Oral Surgery for Dental Students

A Quick Reference Guide

Jeffrey A. Elo, DDS, MS, FACS, FACD, FICD
Professor
Division of Oral and Maxillofacial Surgery
College of Dental Medicine
Western University of Health Sciences
Pomona, California;
Assistant Professor
Department of Oral and Maxillofacial Surgery
Loma Linda University School of Dentistry
Loma Linda, California

Alan S. Herford, DDS, MD, FACS, FACD, FICD
Professor and Chairman
Department of Oral and Maxillofacial Surgery;
Philip J. Boyne and Peter Geistlich Professor
Oral and Maxillofacial Surgery
Loma Linda University School of Dentistry
Loma Linda, California

172 illustrations

Thieme
New York • Stuttgart • Delhi • Rio de Janeiro

Acquisitions Editor: Delia K. DeTurris
Managing Editor: Prakash Naorem
Director, Editorial Services: Mary Jo Casey
Production Editor: Rohit Dev Bhardwaj
International Production Director: Andreas Schabert
Editorial Director: Sue Hodgson
International Marketing Director: Fiona Henderson
International Sales Director: Louisa Turrell
Senior Vice President and Chief Operating
    Officer: Sarah Vanderbilt
President: Brian D. Scanlan

Library of Congress Cataloging-in-Publication Data

Names: Elo, Jeffrey A., editor. | Herford, Alan S., editor.
Title: Oral surgery for dental students : a quick
    reference guide / [edited by] Jeffrey A. Elo, Alan S.
    Herford.
Description: New York : Thieme, [2019] | Includes
    bibliographical references and index. |
Identifiers: LCCN 2019014768 (print) |
    LCCN 2019015662 (ebook) | ISBN 9781626239111 |
    ISBN 9781626239104 (spiral bound) |
    ISBN 9781626239111 (e-book)
Subjects: | MESH: Oral Surgical Procedures
Classification: LCC RK307 (ebook) | LCC RK307 (print) |
    NLM WU 600 | DDC 617.5/22–dc23
LC record available at https://lccn.loc.gov/2019014768

© 2019 Thieme Medical Publishers, Inc.

Thieme Publishers New York
333 Seventh Avenue, New York, NY 10001 USA
+1 800 782 3488, customerservice@thieme.com

Thieme Publishers Stuttgart
Rüdigerstrasse 14, 70469 Stuttgart, Germany
+49 [0]711 8931 421, customerservice@thieme.de

Thieme Publishers Delhi
A-12, Second Floor, Sector-2, Noida-201301
Uttar Pradesh, India
+91 120 45 566 00, customerservice@thieme.in

Thieme Publishers Rio de Janeiro,
Thieme Publicações Ltda.
Edifício Rodolpho de Paoli, 25º andar
Av. Nilo Peçanha, 50 – Sala 2508,
Rio de Janeiro 20020-906 Brasil
+55 21 3172 - 2297

Cover design: Thieme Publishing Group   54321
Typesetting by DiTech Process Solutions, India

Printed in USA by King Printing Company, Inc.

ISBN 978-1-62623-910-4

Also available as an e-book:
eISBN 978-1-62623-911-1

Important note: Medicine is an ever-changing science undergoing continual development. Research and clinical experience are continually expanding our knowledge, in particular our knowledge of proper treatment and drug therapy. Insofar as this book mentions any dosage or application, readers may rest assured that the authors, editors, and publishers have made every effort to ensure that such references are in accordance with **the state of knowledge at the time of production of the book.**

Nevertheless, this does not involve, imply, or express any guarantee or responsibility on the part of the publishers in respect to any dosage instructions and forms of applications stated in the book. **Every user is requested to examine carefully** the manufacturers' leaflets accompanying each drug and to check, if necessary in consultation with a physician or specialist, whether the dosage schedules mentioned therein or the contraindications stated by the manufacturers differ from the statements made in the present book. Such examination is particularly important with drugs that are either rarely used or have been newly released on the market. Every dosage schedule or every form of application used is entirely at the user's own risk and responsibility. The authors and publishers request every user to report to the publishers any discrepancies or inaccuracies noticed. If errors in this work are found after publication, errata will be posted at www.thieme.com on the product description page.

Some of the product names, patents, and registered designs referred to in this book are in fact registered trademarks or proprietary names even though specific reference to this fact is not always made in the text. Therefore, the appearance of a name without designation as proprietary is not to be construed as a representation by the publisher that it is in the public domain.

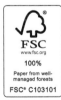

FSC
www.fsc.org
100%
Paper from well-managed forests
FSC® C103101

Contents

Videos

Video 1: Step-by-step extraction of a right maxillary lateral incisor using periotomes and forceps. The video demonstrates proper patient positioning, surgical armamentarium, patient comfort and safety devices, administration of local anesthesia, extraction of the tooth, and suturing the site.

Video 2: Step-by-step extraction of a left maxillary central incisor using periotomes, elevator, and forceps. The video demonstrates proper patient positioning, surgical armamentarium, patient comfort and safety devices, administration of local anesthesia, extraction of the tooth, and suturing the site.

Video 3: Suturing techniques. This 5-minute video demonstrates surgical armamentarium and three commonly used suturing techniques: interrupted suture, continuous suture, and figure-8 suture.

Video 4: Time out procedure. This 1-minute video demonstrates the performance of a time out procedure to verify the correct patient, correct procedure, and correct site for a live patient.

Preface

Oral Surgery for Dental Students: A Quick Reference Guide was developed to provide ready access to essential material and help improve the delivery of basic dental/oral surgery patient care. With a format that allows quick access to key facts, it is our hope that both young and seasoned practitioners alike will now have a go-to "white coat pocket book" that is focused on well-organized, concise, and portable information.

Disclaimer

The information contained in *Oral Surgery for Dental Students: A Quick Reference Guide* is provided as a reference for dental students, recent graduates, and experienced practitioners. The author and contributors do not make any guarantees, expressed or implied, regarding the accuracy and completeness of their products for purposes of clinical treatments. Although the information contained herein has been carefully researched and reviewed for correctness, by utilizing this text, the reader agrees that neither the author nor the contributors accept any legal responsibility for inadvertent errors or omissions that may be present. It is the obligation of every practitioner to review any product or service with regards to the most up-to-date indications, contraindications, dosages, and side effects to ensure safe delivery and use of the products or services provided.

Persons accessing this guide in any published format (paper, electronic, digital, portable electronic device) assume full responsibility for the use of enclosed information and agree that the editors, authors, and contributors are not responsible or liable for any claims, losses, or damages arising from its use or distribution. Any reference to specific products, treatment protocols or processes, resources, web sites, or services does not constitute or imply recommendation or endorsement.

Jeffrey A. Elo, DDS, MS, FACS, FACD, FICD
Alan S. Herford, DDS, MD, FACS, FACD, FICD

Contributors

Elizabeth A. Andrews, DDS, MS
Associate Dean for Academic Affairs
Associate Professor
Division of Oral and Maxillofacial Pathology
College of Dental Medicine
Western University of Health Sciences
Pomona, California

Eric W. Baker, MA, MPhil
Clinical Associate Professor
Director of Head and Neck Anatomy;
Vice-Chair
Department of Basic Science and Craniofacial
    Biology
New York University College of Dentistry
New York, New York

Ronald Caloss, Jr., DDS, MD
Professor
Department of Oral-Maxillofacial Surgery
    and Pathology
School of Dentistry
University of Mississippi Medical Center
Jackson, Mississippi

Vincent Carrao, DDS, MD, FACS
Chief of Oral and Maxillofacial Surgery
Residency Program Director
Division of Oral and Maxillofacial Surgery
Department of Otolaryngology
The Mount Sinai Hospital
Mount Sinai Icahn School of Medicine
New York, New York

**Joseph E. Cillo, Jr., DMD, MPH, PhD, FACS,
    FAACMFS**
Associate Professor of Surgery
Residency Program Director
Director of Research
Drexel University College of Medicine
Division of Oral and Maxillofacial Surgery
Allegheny General Hospital
Allegheny Health Network
Pittsburgh, Pennsylvania

David R. Cummings, DDS, FACD, FICD
Assistant Clinical Professor
Department of Oral and Maxillofacial
    Surgery
Ostrow School of Dentistry
University of Southern California
Los Angeles, California;
Private Practice—OC Centers for Oral Surgery
    and Dental Implants
Orange County, California

Jeffrey A. Elo, DDS, MS, FACS,, FACD, FICD
Professor
Division of Oral and Maxillofacial Surgery
College of Dental Medicine
Western University of Health Sciences
Pomona, California;
Assistant Professor
Department of Oral and Maxillofacial
    Surgery
Loma Linda University School of Dentistry
Loma Linda, California

Steven L. Fletcher, DDS, FACS
Associate Professor
Residency Program Director
Department of Oral and Maxillofacial
Surgery
College of Dentistry
University of Iowa
Iowa City, Iowa

Alan S. Herford, DDS, MD, FACS, FACD, FICD
Professor and Chairman
Department of Oral and Maxillofacial
Surgery;
Philip J. Boyne and Peter Geistlich Professor
Oral and Maxillofacial Surgery
Loma Linda University School of Dentistry
Loma Linda, California

Brett J. King, DDS
Assistant Professor
Department of Oral and Maxillofacial
Surgery
School of Dentistry
Division of Plastic and Reconstructive
Surgery
Department of Surgery
School of Medicine
Louisiana State University Health
Sciences Center
New Orleans, Louisiana

Deepak G. Krishnan, DDS, FACS
Associate Professor of Surgery
Residency Program Director
Division of Oral and Maxillofacial Surgery
University of Cincinnati Medical Center
Cincinnati, Ohio

Edward T. Lahey, DMD, MD, FACS
Assistant Professor
Department of Oral and Maxillofacial
Surgery
Harvard School of Dental Medicine
Medical Director
Quality and Safety Chair
Department of Oral and Maxillofacial
Surgery
Massachusetts General Hospital
Boston, Massachusetts

Setareh Lavasani, DDS, MS, FGDIA
Assistant Professor
Director of Oral Radiology and Advanced
Imaging
Division of Oral and Maxillofacial Radiology
College of Dental Medicine
Western University of Health Sciences
Pomona, California

Julie O'Meara, BDS, BMedSci
Adjunct Instructor
Department of Basic Science and Craniofacial
Biology
New York University College of Dentistry
New York, New York

Chan M. Park, DDS, MD, FACS
Division Chief and Program Director
Division of Oral and Maxillofacial Surgery
Alameda Health System, Highland Hospital
Oakland, California;
Associate Professor
University of the Pacific, Dugoni School of
Dentistry
San Francisco, California

Riddhi Patel, DMD
Clinical Instructor of Surgery
Division of Oral and Maxillofacial Surgery
Department of Surgery
University of Cincinnati
Cincinnati, Ohio

Rawle F. Philbert, DDS, FACD
Chair and OMS Residency Program Director
Department of Dentistry/Oral and
    Maxillofacial Surgery
Lincoln Medical and Mental Health Center
Bronx, New York;
Clinical Associate Professor
Department of Oral and Maxillofacial
    Surgery
College of Dental Medicine
Columbia University
New York, New York;
Clinical Assistant Professor
Department of Surgery
Weil Cornell Medical School
New York, New York

Benjamin R. Shimel, DDS
Assistant Program Director
Division of Oral and Maxillofacial Surgery
Alameda Health System, Highland Hospital
Oakland, California;
Assistant Professor
University of the Pacific, Dugoni School of
    Dentistry
San Francisco, California

Ho-Hyun Sun, DMD, MS
Resident
Division of Oral and Maxillofacial Surgery
Alameda Health System, Highland Hospital
Oakland, California;
University of the Pacific, Dugoni School of
    Dentistry
San Francisco, California

Christopher F. Viozzi, MD, DDS
Consultant in Surgery
Assistant Professor of Surgery
Mayo Clinic
Rochester, Minnesota

Christopher H. Yi, BS
Senior Dental Student
College of Dental Medicine
Western University of Health Sciences
Pomona, California

1 New Patient Visit

Jeffrey A. Elo, Alan S. Herford, Ho-Hyun Sun, Christopher H. Yi

Consultation Visit—New Patient Script

One of the greatest sources of anxiety and confusion for preclinical and new-to-clinic dental students is *What should I say to the patient*? Learning *what* to say and *how* to say it to patients is an important skill worthy of development. Of course, it takes time to get the words, rhythm, and the delivery correct, but doing so may help the practitioner appear friendly, amicable, and thorough while instilling confidence in the listening patient. But importantly, this must occur within a short period of time.

Over the years, many generations of students and young practitioners have found it immensely helpful to have some *scripts*—well-practiced guidelines—as far as what to say, how to say, and what level of depth to delve into when first interacting with patients. Good practitioners work at fine-tuning their delivery when it comes to greeting a new patient, discussing their findings/diagnoses, presenting the treatment plan, and then closing out the visit.

This is meant to be a starting point for new practitioners or those with high anxiety about the first few times when they have a patient in their chair.

Example: The following might be a sample consultation *script* to use as a guideline when meeting a new patient "Ms. Jones" who has a painful, nonrestorable mandibular molar that requires removal.

"Good morning, Ms. Jones, my name is (student) Doctor_____. Tell me what brings you in today. I understand that you have a broken molar causing you pain, and that you would like to have it removed. Is that correct? We are more than happy to get that taken care of for you. First, let me ask you a couple of questions. Do you have any medical conditions or concerns that you are currently being treated for, such as diabetes or asthma? Do you have any problems with your heart or with high blood pressure? Do you get pains in your chest or lose your breath when walking or doing any form of activity, or even from just sitting? Have you had any issues with bleeding in the past? Are you currently taking any prescription or nonprescription medications? Do you have any allergies to any medications—penicillin, codeine, or dental numbing medicine? Do you smoke? If so, how much and for how many years? Do you drink alcohol? Do you use any other recreational drugs—marijuana, cocaine, or heroin? It is important for us to know these things because some of our medications or treatments might interact with certain drugs or chemicals. Have you had any surgeries in the past? Have you ever had any problems with anesthesia that you know of or were told about? Have you ever had any problems with local anesthesia in a dental office? What we will do right now is take a look at your radiograph(s), talk about what we see and what we can offer you, and then we'll leave any decision-making up to you. Okay?"

When reviewing diagnostic material such as a panoramic radiograph, a thorough, verbal description in terms understandable to the patient is helpful. You can say something like the following (while using your hands or a pointer to describe as you speak).

"In the radiograph(s), these teeth up here (indicating with a pointer) are your top teeth; these are your bottom teeth. This is your right side; this is your left side. Let us zoom in on the bad molar causing your pain. This tooth is missing tooth structure and has a deep cavity, or a hole, that we can see in this dark area of the tooth. Notice how it appears very different in color from the other surrounding teeth.

Because of how much tooth structure is missing, we are not able to fix that with our dental techniques. The only treatment we can offer you is removal or extraction. Most patients do well with these procedures with local anesthesia—where we give you some numbing medicine in the area so you do not feel any pain. You will feel pressure as I am working, but there will be no discomfort or pain. You might even hear some funny noises as we are working, but that is normal, as well. We might have to make a small incision in the gums. If we do, it will only be as long as the tooth from front to back, so it will not be very big. But that will allow us better access to the entire tooth so we can work more quickly and get you back on your way. Once we get the tooth out, we will put in some dissolvable stitches to close the gums. This also helps with the healing process. The procedure will take about 10 to 20 minutes once you are numb and comfortable. And after we are done you will be ready to go home.

Then comes your recovery phase. It is normal and expected for some swelling to occur. It takes about 3 days for this swelling to reach its peak before it starts to get better. There also is a possibility of bruising in the area. Bruising typically lasts longer than swelling, but it will go away. There are no diet restrictions or activity restrictions. You can eat and drink whatever is comfortable for you, but perhaps it will be wise to stay away from sharper-edged foods, such as chips, for a few days. And lastly, we will be giving you two or three medication prescriptions to take during your recovery. One is a pain medication such as acetaminophen (Tylenol®). Take it if you need it. One is a medicated mouthwash. It is like a topical antibiotic and helps the gum tissue and the socket heal more quickly. And the last one is something like Motrin® or Advil® that helps minimize your swelling and contributes to pain relief.

Let me discuss with you the risks of the procedure. The main risks of any tooth removal procedure are some minor discomfort, swelling, and bleeding or oozing following surgery. These are all normal and expected. There is a low risk of infection, but these are rare. There is also a small possibility that additional surgery may be needed if the site fails to heal properly. It is unlikely, but adjacent teeth or nerve structures can be bruised, bumped, or nicked during the process of completing our work. We will make every effort to avoid this, but it is possible. There is also a chance that we may decide to leave a small piece of the tooth or root behind if attempting to remove it places important structures, such as nerves, at risk of injury or damage. We will discuss this, if needed, during the procedure so you are fully aware of what is happening and why.

The benefits of this treatment include removing the bad tooth that is the source of your pain. After a brief healing period of a couple days, you should be feeling a lot better.

The only alternative treatment option is to not remove the tooth and leave it in, as is. However, leaving that tooth in will continue to cause you pain and put you at risk for continued or worsening infection. Root canal therapy is not an option because there is too much tooth destruction from the large cavity.

Do you have any questions?

I am going to go ahead and enter a treatment plan, which is just a list of the procedure(s) we talked about. One of our staff members will go over the treatment plan, have you sign the plan if you are in agreement, and take you to the scheduler who can get you scheduled for an appointment. There is also a procedure consent form we will need to have you sign.

We will take very good care of you, okay."

Typically, the above conversation and guided questioning can be done in about 10 minutes. The script is direct and focused, and guides the young practitioner to stay efficient and on topic with their time. By maintaining direction and focus in the consultation, the practitioner can maximize each patient's chair time. Practicing this as a student doctor will enable the graduate to be highly skilled in the art of patient communication by the time he/she is ready to see many more patients in private practice.

Consultation Talking Points

Efficiency is most easily achieved through repetition. Below is a list of talking points that should be mentioned during a consultation. Practice implementing this list into a personalized script. This is merely a suggested order and all providers should make their own list. However, delivery should be made in the same sequence each time so that key elements are not omitted.

1. Introduce yourself and establish patient rapport.
2. Review patients' chief complaint and what brings them in.
3. Review medical history, past surgeries, and conditions.
4. Review list of medications and allergies.
5. Note past anesthesia issues.
6. Review radiographs.
7. Explain procedure: include specific preop instructions if needed, time frame, as well as postop expectations.
8. Answer questions, if any.
9. Review treatment plan, consent, and next step(s).

Charts and Charting

- Most attorneys say that if something is not written in the chart, it did not happen.
- Document every encounter with patients.
- If you call a patient, document it in the chart.
- If you see a patient, document the progress notes in the chart.
- If you are scheduled to see a patient, and he/she fails to show, document it.

Comprehensive Oral Evaluation—History and Physical Examination

- A thorough medical history and complete head and neck physical examination should be performed for every *new* patient and on yearly or semiannual reevaluation visits.
- It should include the following items:
    - Identification [ID] (*age, race, gender*).
    - Chief complaint [CC] (*why is the patient here?*).
    - History of the present illness [HPI] (*how long has the problem been going on?*).
    - Past medical history [PMH] (include primary care physician's name and phone number, current illnesses, and past illnesses or hospitalizations).
    - Past surgical history (PSH).
    - Social history (Soc).
        - *Tobacco use*: pack years = packs per day × number of years smoked.
        - *Alcohol use* (type, amount, frequency).
        - *Recreational drug use* (specify the drug and route).
    - Medications [Meds] (*prescription and nonprescription*).
    - Allergies (ALL).
    - American Society of Anesthesiologists' (ASA) status.

Physical Exam

- Vital signs.
    - Blood pressure (BP).
    - Heart rate (HR).
    - Temperature (T).
    - Respiratory rate (RR).
- General.
    - Height.
    - Weight.
    - Body mass index (BMI).

- Facial skin.
  - Visible rashes.
  - Lesions.
  - Scars.
  - Tattoos.
- Oral cavity.
  - Occlusion and dental condition.
  - Also evaluate the following for presence of any abnormalities:
    - Tongue.
    - Floor of mouth.
    - Buccal mucosa/vestibule.
    - Lips.
    - Hard/soft palate.
    - Tonsils.
    - Oropharynx.
- Neck.
  - Lymphadenopathy (LAD).
  - Thyroid size.
  - Jugular venous distention (JVD).

Radiographic Findings

- Any abnormalities seen on radiographs (see Chapter 5, Essentials of Dental Radiographic Analysis and Interpretation).

Assessment

- Diagnoses or a list of issues.

Plan

- Suggested course of treatment action.

Comprehensive Oral Evaluation on New Patient—Sample Note

Meticulous record-keeping and note-taking is essential for successful dental practice. Undocumented discussions are not considered in a court of law.

A complete sample consultation note for a new patient exam should be written in a manner similar to the following:

ID/CC: A 42-year-old female presents for removal of her symptomatic, fractured, carious, nonrestorable tooth number 19.

HPI: Patient reports that this tooth broke about 2 months ago while eating popcorn. She has been having intermittent pain ever since.

PMH: Hypothyroidism, iron-deficiency anemia.

PSH: Gallbladder removal 3 years prior—no anesthetic complications.

Soc: Half pack per day cigarette use × 10 years (five pack year history); occasional beer drinker; no hard liquor; smokes marijuana five times per week.

Meds: Levothyroxine, iron supplement.

ALL: Penicillin—rash.

ASA: 2

Exam: BP: 115/75 (right arm, sitting); HR: 68; T: 98.7; RR: 15.

Height: 5′1″.

Weight: 115 lb.

BMI: 21.7.

Extraoral/ facial skin: No visible rashes, lesions, scars, or tattoos; maximum interincisal opening of 35 mm, cranial nerves V2 and V3 grossly intact bilaterally, right temporomandibular joint (TMJ) reciprocal click with no pain.

Oral cavity: Class 1 molar/canine relationship with some anterior dental crowding/malpositioning; right anterior dorsum of tongue with 5 mm firm fibroma-like lesion; buccal mucosa with linea alba noted bilaterally; vestibule, lips, hard/soft palate, tonsils, and oropharynx with no apparent lesions or ulcerations; tooth number 19 is fractured with exposed pulp and missing coronal tooth structure—nonrestorable.

Neck: Left submandibular LAD—one pea-sized node noted that is freely movable and tender to palpation.

X-rays: Panoramic radiograph shows fractured tooth number 19 with 3 mm periapical radiolucency on mesial root apex.

Assessment: Fractured, carious, nonrestorable tooth number 19.

Plan: Local anesthesia, surgical extraction of tooth number 19, excisional biopsy of periapical lesion with submission to oral pathologist, placement of mineralized allograft to site number 19. Anticipate 45 minutes of chair time.

Risks/benefits/alternatives discussed with patient in detail; all questions were answered to patient's satisfaction; treatment plan and consent forms signed.

Surgical Treatment Note—Sample Note

The 42-year-old female returned to clinic for local anesthesia, removal of nonrestorable, carious tooth number 19, excisional biopsy of periapical lesion, socket allograft; procedure and consent reviewed/signature verified. "Time out" procedure was performed prior to the administration of local anesthetic.

Preop BP: 118/76, P: 78.

Treatment: 1.7 mL of 2% lidocaine with 1:100k epi given as left inferior alveolar nerve (IAN) block; 1.0 mL of 2% lidocaine with 1:100k epi given as left long buccal infiltration; crestal incision on facial surface of tooth number 19 created with number 15 blade; full thickness flap elevated on facial surface of tooth number 19; surgical hand piece used to incompletely section tooth number 19 into mesial and distal roots; Bayonet elevator used to complete sectioning and deliver the distal root; number 190 elevator used to deliver mesial root; curette used to excise mesial root periapical granuloma/cyst which was then placed in formalin, bone file used to smooth facial bone; copious saline irrigation of socket and under facial flap; placed 0.7 mL mineralized allograft to socket number 19; 3-0 chromic gut continuous sutures placed from mesial papilla to distal papilla; hemostasis achieved; patient tolerated very well. Tissue specimen will be submitted to oral pathology laboratory.

Postop BP: 121/82, P: 71.

Prescriptions given: Ibuprofen 600 mg, #12 tabs, 1 tab PO q6h prn pain; acetaminophen 500 mg, #12 tabs, 1 tab PO q6h prn pain; chlorhexidine gluconate 0.12%, 1 bottle, 15 cc PO swish 30 second/spit tid til gone.

Postop instructions sheet given and reviewed verbally with patient.

Next visit: Follow-up in 1 to 2 weeks for postop check, or as needed.

Clinical Pearls
- Make sure to call patients in the evening following a procedure.
- Even if the procedure was not a "big deal" for you to perform, it most certainly is a big deal from the patient's standpoint.
- They will appreciate the call and may have questions about their postop care or prescriptions.

Limited Oral Evaluation—Sample Consultation Note

ID/CC: 18-year-old female presents for evaluation regarding removal of her symptomatic, grossly carious, nonrestorable upper right first molar tooth number 3.

HPI: She reports intermittent pain, swelling, and drainage associated with this tooth.

PMH: Exercise-induced asthma; no hospitalizations or emergency room visits in the last 5 years for asthma-related illness; uses rescue inhaler as needed; typical trigger for asthma attacks includes running more than a block in cold weather; denies history of heart, liver, kidney, bleeding, infectious, or other disorders.

PSH: Appendix removal 3 years ago—no general anesthetic or surgical complications.

Soc: Tobacco/cigarette use—half pack per day × 2 years; denies alcohol use; reports marijuana use 1 to 2 times per week; denies any other recreational drug use.

Meds: Albuterol MDI as needed for asthma/wheezing (1 time per month typically).

ALL: Penicillin—reports getting a rash.

Exam: Well developed, well nourished; head, eyes, ears, and nose exam unremarkable; maximum interincisal opening 35 mm, cranial nerves V2 and V3 intact bilaterally; remaining cranial nerves grossly intact; neck is supple with no masses, thyroid swellings, or LAD noted; full adult dentition; fair oral hygiene; oropharynx clear; grossly carious, fractured, nonrestorable tooth number 3; all other oral hard and soft tissues appear normal.

X-rays: Panoramic radiograph and periapical radiograph reveal a grossly carious, fractured, nonrestorable tooth number 3; also noted are mesially tipped, full bony impacted teeth numbers 17 and 32, along with vertically positioned, partial bony impacted teeth numbers 1 and 16.

Assessment: Grossly carious, fractured, nonrestorable tooth number 3.

Plan: Local anesthesia, surgical extraction of tooth number 3. Anticipate 30 minutes of chair time.

Risks/benefits/alternatives discussed with patient (guardian if a minor) in detail; all questions were answered to patient's satisfaction; treatment plan and consent forms signed.

Medical Consultation Request

Some patients are either poor medical historians or erroneously report several medical conditions or illnesses. These individuals may not recall their complete medical or surgical histories or realize the current status of their current health conditions. Some patients might be good historians but possess complicated histories that require elaboration. For either of these reasons, or at any time a provider feels the need to obtain additional information regarding the patient's health status, a medical consultation request may be made.

A simple phone call to the patient's physician may provide answers to the clinician's dilemma of "Should I treat this patient?" The dental provider must recognize when and for which patients more information should be obtained. Some examples might include:

- Recent surgery or hospitalization.
- History of chest pain, heart attack, or stroke.
- Diabetic management.
- Chronic kidney or liver disease/failure.
- Lung diseases such as asthma or chronic obstructive pulmonary disease (COPD).
- Allergies/drug reactions.

The commonly used phrase *Medical Clearance* is no longer recommended, as medical physicians cannot provide *clearance* for any particular dental procedure. However, they may be able to provide a list of the patient's current medical diagnoses/conditions and the status of their management. After consulting with the physician, a dental practitioner may formulate a treatment plan to best manage their mutual patient.

Sample Medical Consultation Request Letter

Date

Primary Care Doctor Name
Primary Care Doctor Address
Primary Care Doctor Phone

Re: Patient Name
Patient Date of Birth (DOB)

Dear Primary Care Doctor,

Today, I had the pleasure of meeting with Mr. Patient Name. He was referred to us for evaluation for removal of his remaining maxillary and mandibular teeth (20 teeth total) in preparation for immediate delivery of new complete dentures.

9

PMH: Hepatitis C, diabetes mellitus type 2, severe dental anxiety, hypothyroidism, diabetic neuropathy, hypercholesterolemia, depression, hypertension—poorly controlled.

PSH: Gallbladder removal 2 years ago.

Soc: History of methamphetamine and heroin use—quit 2 years ago; none currently.

Meds: Atorvastatin, gabapentin, levothyroxine, fenofibrate, metformin, sertraline, lisinopril, ASA 81 mg, amlodipine.

ALL: No known drug allergies.

Exam: Clinical and radiographic evaluation revealed nonrestorable maxillary and mandibular teeth, along with irregular alveolar ridges in the upper and lower arches.

My recommendations: In consideration of his complex medical history and the amount of surgery required to properly treat Mr. Patient Name, I want to ensure that Patient Name does not have any significant bleeding risk. We plan on performing his surgery in two stages under local anesthesia (2% lidocaine with 1:100k epinephrine) in the clinic.

I am asking for you to order and provide for me the following laboratory studies:

1. Prothrombin time (PT).
2. International normalized ratio (INR).
3. Complete blood count.
4. HbA1c.
5. Recent history and physical exam with current status of each medical condition.

Thank you, in advance, for your assistance in facilitating the care of Mr. Patient Name. If you should have any questions regarding the care of this patient, please feel free to give me a call.

Sincerely,
Dental Provider Name
Dental Provider Title
Dental Provider Address
Phone: 800.123.4567
Fax: 800.890.1234

American Society of Anesthesiologists' (ASA) Physical Status Classification

ASA physical status classification	Definition	Examples, including, but not limited to:
ASA I	A normal healthy patient	Healthy, nonsmoking, no or minimal alcohol use
ASA II	A patient with mild systemic disease	Mild diseases only without substantive functional limitations. Examples include (but not limited to): current smoker, social alcohol drinker, pregnancy, obesity (30 < BMI < 40), well-controlled DM/HTN, mild lung disease
ASA III	A patient with severe systemic disease	Substantive functional limitations; one or more moderate to severe diseases. Examples include (but not limited to): poorly controlled DM or HTN, COPD, morbid obesity (BMI ≥ 40), active hepatitis, alcohol dependence or abuse, implanted pacemaker, moderate reduction of ejection fraction, ESRD undergoing regularly scheduled dialysis, premature infant PCA < 60 weeks, history (> 3 months) of MI, CVA, TIA, or CAD/stents
ASA IV	A patient with severe systemic disease that is a constant threat to life	Examples include (but not limited to): recent (< 3 months) MI, CVA, TIA, or CAD/stents, ongoing cardiac ischemia or severe valve dysfunction, severe reduction of ejection fraction, sepsis, DIC, ARD or ESRD not undergoing regularly scheduled dialysis
ASA V	A moribund patient who is not expected to survive without the operation	Examples include (but not limited to): ruptured abdominal/thoracic aneurysm, massive trauma, intracranial bleed with mass effect, ischemic bowel in the face of significant cardiac pathology or multiple organ/system dysfunction
ASA VI	A declared brain-dead patient whose organs are being removed for donor purposes	

Note: The addition of "E" denoted emergency surgery: an emergency is defined as existing when delay in treatment of the patient would lead to a significant increase in the threat to life or body part.

Abbreviations: ARDS, acute respiratory distress syndrome; BMI, body mass index; CAD, coronary artery disease; COPD, chronic obstructive pulmonary disease; CVA, cerebrovascular accident; DIC, disseminated intravascular coagulation; DM, diabetes mellitus; ESRD, end-stage renal disease; HTN, hypertension; MI, myocardial infarction; PCA, post conceptual age; TIA, transient ischemic attack. (Adapted from https://www.asahq.org/resources/clinical-information/asa-physical-status-classification-system.)

Antibiotic Prophylaxis Prior to Dental Procedures

- Prosthetic joints.
  - A January 2015 ADA clinical practice guideline—based on a 2014 systematic review—does not recommend prophylactic antibiotics for patients with prosthetic joint implants prior to dental procedures.

Antibiotic Prophylaxis Prior to Dental Procedures

- Infective endocarditis (IE).
  - IE is much more likely to result from frequent exposure to random bacteremias associated with daily activities than from bacteremia caused by a dental procedure.
  - Prophylaxis may prevent an exceedingly small number of cases of IE, if any, in people who undergo dental procedures.
  - The risk of antibiotic-associated adverse events exceeds the benefit, if any, from prophylactic antibiotic therapy.
  - Maintenance of optimal oral health and hygiene may reduce the incidence of bacteremia from daily activities and is more important than prophylactic antibiotics for a dental procedure to reduce the risk of IE.

Cardiac conditions associated with the highest risk of adverse outcome from endocarditis for which prophylaxis with dental procedures is reasonable

- Prosthetic cardiac valve or prosthetic material used for cardiac valve repair.
- Previous infective endocarditis.
- Congenital heart disease (CHD)[a]
- Unrepaired cyanotic CHD, including palliative shunts and conduits.
- Completely repaired CHD with prosthetic material or device, whether placed by surgery or by catheter intervention, during the first 6 months after the procedure.[b]
- Repaired CHD with residual defects at the site or adjacent to the site of a prosthetic patch or prosthetic device (which inhibit endothelialization).
- Cardiac transplantation recipients who develop cardiac valvulopathy.

[a]Except for the conditions listed above, antibiotic prophylaxis is no longer recommended for any other form of CHD.
[b]Prophylaxis is reasonable because endothelialization of prosthetic material occurs within 6 months after the procedure.
Source: Wilson W, et al. Prevention of infective endocarditis: guidelines from the American Heart Association. JADA. 2008;139:3S–24S.

Dental procedures for which endocarditis prophylaxis is reasonable

All dental procedures that involve manipulation of gingival tissue or the periapical region of teeth or perforation of the oral mucosa.[a]

[a]The following procedures and events do not need prophylaxis: routine anesthetic injections through noninfected tissue, taking dental radiographs, placement of removable prosthodontic or orthodontic appliances, adjustment of orthodontic appliances, placement of orthodontic brackets, shedding of primary teeth, and bleeding from trauma to the lips or oral mucosa.

▶ Table 1.1 displays the American Heart Association prophylactic antibiotic guideline regimens for a dental procedure.

Table 1.1 Prophylactic antibiotic regimens for a dental procedure

Situation	Agent	Regimen: single dose 30–60 minutes before procedure	
		Adults	Children
Oral	Amoxicillin	2 g	50 mg/kg
Unable to take oral medication	Ampicillin OR	2 g IM or IV	50 mg/kg IM or IV
	cefazolin or ceftriaxone	1 g IM or IV	50 mg/kg IM or IV
Allergic to penicillins or ampicillin	Cephalexin[a,b] OR	2g	50 mg/kg
	clindamycin OR	600 mg	20 mg/kg
	azithromycin or clarithromycin	500 mg	15 mg/kg
Allergic to penicillins or ampicillin and unable to take oral medication	Cefazolin or ceftriaxone[b] OR	1 g IM or IV	50 mg/kg IM or IV
	clindamycin	600 mg IM or IV	20 mg/kg IM or IV

Abbreviations: IM, intramuscular; IV, intravenous.
[a]Or other first- or second-generation oral cephalosporin in equivalent adult or pediatric dosage.
[b]Cephalosporins should not be used in a person with a history of anaphylaxis, angioedema, or urticaria with penicillins or ampicillin.

Source: Wilson W, Taubert KA, Gewitz M, et al. Prevention of infective endocarditis: guidelines from the American Heart Association. Circulation. 2007;116:1736–1754.

13

2 Infection Control

Joseph E. Cillo, Jr., Jeffrey A. Elo, Alan S. Herford

Personal Protective Equipment

- Protective gown or apron.
- Gloves.
- Facemask with/without shield.
- Protective eyewear.
- Long hair should be tied back or placed under a hair covering.
- No dangling earrings.
- Jewelry should be avoided.
- Bare below the elbows.

Infection Control

- Practice proper hand hygiene:
  - Wash hands adequately before and after treating patients.
    - Alcohol.
    - Hand sanitizers.
    - Soap.
  - Avoid rings and long or acrylic fingernails as they can trap dirt, debris, and bacteria.
  - Jewelry can tear through protective gloves and promote contamination.
  - Glove types determine potential contact dermatitis/latex sensitivity. Following types of gloves are used:
    - Utility gloves.
    - Nitrile gloves.
    - Sterile surgery gloves.
    - Overgloves.
  - Avoid unnecessary contact with used gloves to avoid cross contamination.
  - Change gloves frequently, especially when they are visibly soiled.
- Surface disinfection:
  - Follow appropriate directions when using disinfectant wipes or solutions.
  - Allow sufficient surface contact time:
    - Avoid wiping away the cleaner prematurely.
  - Clean surfaces to remove debris before disinfection:
    - Preclean before disinfecting.
  - Use Environmental Protection Agency (EPA)-registered hospital-grade disinfectants.
- Barriers:
  - Barriers must be replaced between patients.

- Effective instrument processing:
  - Clean the instruments first to remove visible debris.
  - Avoid banding instruments together or overloading the ultrasonic tank.
    - Allow full penetration of the ultrasonic solution and its activity to all surfaces of the instruments.
  - Avoid using dish soap or cold sterile solution instead of ultrasonic solution.
- Proper instrument wrapping:
  - Use the correct type of wrap or packaging material.
  - Seal the wraps or pouches correctly.
  - Do not place too many instruments in the wrap or pouch.
  - Dry the instruments before wrapping.
- Avoid sterilization pit falls:
  - Allow adequate time for the cycle to run and be completed.
  - Ensure appropriate sterilization temperature and pressure.
  - Adequately preclean the instruments prior to sterilization.
  - Do not overload the sterilizer.
  - Ensure an adequate drying cycle for autoclaves.
  - Ensure that the gaskets and seals are effective.
  - Avoid bulky or improper packaging.
  - Ensure adequate spacing of instrument packets.
  - Periodically test and ensure proper operation of the sterilization unit.
  - Use the correct type of sterilization packaging material to achieve desired sterilization.
    - Some materials may prevent the sterilizing agent from reaching inside the instruments.
    - Certain plastics may melt.
    - Paper products may burn or char.
    - Thick cloths may unnecessarily retain steam or chemical vapor.
    - Closed containers are not appropriate for steam or unsaturated chemical vapor sterilizers.
    - Lint fibers may cause postoperative complications and serve as vehicles for microorganisms, increasing the risk of infection for surgical patients.
  - Avoid sterilization of unwrapped instruments.
  - An unwrapped cycle, sometimes called a flash sterilization, is a method of sterilizing unwrapped patient-care items for immediate use.
  - Unwrapped sterilization should be used only in cases when:
    - Thorough cleaning and drying of instruments precedes the unwrapped sterilization cycle.
    - Mechanical monitors are checked and chemical indicators are used for each cycle.
    - Care is taken to avoid thermal injury to dental workers or patients.
    - Items are transported aseptically to the treatment site to maintain sterility.

- Avoid malfunctioning sterilizers:
  - Perform spore testing weekly.
  - Service the sterilization unit according to the manufacturer's recommendations.
  - Ensure proper voltage for the unit.
  - Use distilled water for autoclaves.
- Treat dental unit water lines:
  - Flush water lines between each patient.
  - Perform periodic testing of water lines to monitor safe water quality.
  - Use sterile water delivery systems for surgical procedures (sterile saline or sterile water).
- Ensure that single-use disposable items are only used for a single visit.
  - Saliva ejectors.
  - Evacuation tips.
  - Disposable air/water syringe tips.
  - Paper/plastic sterilization pouches or wraps.
  - Any other item intended for single use.

Written Protocol for Operatory Cleanliness

Infection Control Protocol for Operatory Set-Up

- Perform hand hygiene.
- Place environmental barriers.
- Ensure engineering controls are available or are in place.
- Ensure quality treatment water is available.
- Place the patient chart and radiographs in an appropriate visible location.
- Access digital radiographs, if computerized.
- Remove all other excess items from the countertops if not necessary for patient care.
- Ensure that any necessary items received from the dental laboratory have been decontaminated.
- Obtain the instrument packages, trays/cassettes, equipment, and supplies necessary for the appointment.
- Seat the patient and give them protective eye glasses and place the patient napkin/towel.
- Open cassettes or gently spill the instrument packages onto a sterile surface without touching the contents.
- Put on your mask and then your protective eyewear or face shield.
- Wash your hands or use an alcohol hand rub and put on gloves.
- Connect high volume evacuator and saliva ejector tips.

- At the beginning of each workday, dental unit lines shall be purged with air or flushed with water for at least 2 minutes prior to attaching handpieces or other devices.
- The dental unit line shall be flushed between each patient for a minimum of 20 seconds.

Infection Control Protocol for Operatory Clean Up

- While still wearing personal protective equipment, flush dental unit lines for 20 to 30 seconds (air/water syringes, handpieces, and scalers).
- Remove and discard any environmental barriers.
- Place instruments back in the tray or cassette.
- Place all disposable sharps in the sharps container.
- Place unsharp disposable items in a plastic-lined waste container.
- Clean and disinfect all clinical contact surfaces that are not protected by impervious barriers using an EPA-registered, hospital-grade low- to intermediate-level disinfectant after each patient.
- The low-level disinfectants used shall be labeled effective against hepatitis B virus (HBV) and human immunodeficiency virus (HIV).
- Use disinfectants in accordance with the manufacturer's instructions.
- Clean all housekeeping surfaces (e.g., floors, walls, sinks) with a detergent and water, or EPA-registered hospital-grade disinfectant.
- Transport instruments and handpieces to the decontamination/sterilization area.
- Rinse and disinfect any impressions or prosthetic items before taking them into the in-office/clinic lab.
- Remove and decontaminate the eyewear.
- Remove gloves and other protective attire.
- Perform hand hygiene.

Bibliography

[1] Kohn WG, Collins AS, Cleveland JL, Harte JA, Eklund KJ, Malvitz DM, Centers for Disease Control and Prevention (CDC). Guidelines for infection control in dental health-care settings—2003. MMWR Recomm Rep. 2003; 52 RR-17:1–61

[2] Organization for Safety & Asepsis Procedures. Centers for Disease Control and Prevention (U.S.). From policy to practice: OSAP's guide to the guidelines: your tool for applying CDC dental infection control guidelines. Annapolis, MD: OSAP; 2004

3 Time Out Policy: Correct Patient, Correct Procedure, Correct Site

Deepak G. Krishnan, Riddhi Patel, Jeffrey A. Elo

Verification Process Policy

- One of the most common reasons why patients engage in lawsuits against dentists is extraction of the wrong tooth.
- This is a preventable occurrence that often occurs as a result of haste or inattention.
- A "time out" is an opportunity for the dental team to pause and eliminate errors before the treatment begins.

Correct Site Surgery and Time Out Procedure

- Removal of the wrong tooth is a preventable error.
- It represents 10 to 15% of claims in the past 15 years.
- Nearly 50% of claims are settled "no contest."
- Cases are often indefensible because they are typically considered preventable.
- Wrong tooth extractions represent a large outlay in claims, i.e., in dollars.
  - An average of $1,500,000 per year over the past 10 years.
- Wrong tooth extractions can lead to a loss of rapport with patients and colleague dentists.

Replacing Risky Habits with Safer Habits

- Implement a "time out" procedure prior to performing the surgery.
  - It enables the provider to check and verify documentation.
  - It also enables the provider to confirm the following:
    - Correct patient.
    - Correct procedure.
    - Correct site.

Time Out Procedure

- Before the procedure is started, the treatment team pauses to review documentation for the patient identity, procedure, and site.
- If any disparities are encountered, appropriate calls are made and documented prior to the start of the procedure.
- If the disparity cannot be resolved, the procedure is deferred to another time.

EXTRACT: Acronym to Prevent Wrong Tooth Extractions

- **E**xamination: should be independent of the referral doctor's examination and preferably at a separate preoperative consultation appointment.
- **X**-ray check: current and diagnostic; correct patient and spatial orientation.
- **T**reatment plan: does the treatment plan correspond with the referring doctor's?
- **R**eview: chart review preoperatively in advance of the procedure.
- **A**nnounce: current plan with the "time out" procedure.
- **C**ount: the teeth; the first tooth count during the "time out."
- **T**reat: beginning the surgery with a second tooth count.

E: Examination

- It should be independent of the referral doctor's examination and preferably at a separate preoperative consultation appointment.
- Perform an additional clinical and radiographic examination.
- Consultation visit—why it is required?
  - To establish an independent diagnosis.
  - To verify accuracy of the referral.
  - To review medical history in advance of procedure.
  - To consult with the patient's physician if indicated.
  - To review the surgery with the patient (or guardian) when the patient is not premedicated.
  - To make financial arrangements prior to the day of the procedure.
  - To verify insurance benefits/preauthorization.
  - To meet the patient so that he/she is no more a "stranger."
- Without a prior, separate consultation appointment, it is imperative that the office protocols be monitored much more closely on the day of the procedure.

X: X-ray Evaluation

- Following points about radiographs should be taken care of:
  - Are the radiographs of the correct patient?
  - Are they diagnostic?
    - Do they show the procedural area(s)?
  - Are they current?
    - Have they been taken within the last year?
    - Do they reveal the *current condition* of the mouth/teeth?
  - Are they correctly oriented?
    - Right versus left.

19

- At the consultation appointment, identify to the patient the tooth to be extracted.
- Verify the correct radiograph and markings at the time of the procedure.

T: Treatment Plan

- After conducting an independent examination and comparing it to the referral dentist's notes, does the requested treatment on the referral seem reasonable?
- Always take a history and perform a physical examination of your patient.
- Do not depend solely on the examination or history performed by another dentist.
- Consider your state laws regarding record-keeping and note documentation.
  - For example, a California Health and Safety Code states that "a dentist licensed pursuant to Chapter 4…of the business and professional code…" must maintain patient records relating to:
    ○ Health history.
    ○ Diagnosis or condition(s) of a patient.
    ○ Treatment provided or proposed to be provided to the patient.
  - Document following important items:
    ○ Chief complaint.
    ○ History of present illness.
    ○ Clinical findings.

R: Review Chart

- Review the chart preoperatively to assure that there are no problems such as missing notes, referral slips, or radiographs.
- Preoperative chart review:
  - When the chart is reviewed days prior to the procedure, incomplete records, errors, etc. can be noted and corrected.
  - Since the check is conducted days prior to the procedure, there is sufficient time to correct most, if not all, inaccuracies.
  - If the inaccuracy cannot be corrected, there is then still time to reschedule the patient and fill his/her appointment slot with another appointment.
- A preop checklist for all the things to have ready on the day of surgery can be helpful: (*this is the first way that the staff can also help in preventing mistakes.*)
  - Radiograph with correct patient name and date of birth (DOB) or chart number.
    ○ There may be more than one patient with the same name.
    ○ Using the patient's DOB or chart number provides a second method of identification.
  - Referral slip, if present.

– Treatment plan signed and dated.
– Consent form signed and dated.
– Financial arrangement signed and dated.

A: Announce Your Plan

- Conduct a preoperative "time out" to announce the treatment plan to the patient and staff members (*this is the second way the staff can help in preventing mistakes.*)
- Demonstrate which tooth or teeth will undergo extraction.
- The provider, together with the staff and patient, discusses the critical aspects of the upcoming procedure such as the referral, radiograph, treatment plan, medical history, allergies, and consent.
- If a referral slip is present and applicable to the patient, it should be left in direct view of the provider and staff so that the team can readily make note before instruments are placed in the mouth.

C: Count the Teeth

- The first tooth count should be performed along with the time out so that the provider, staff, and patient are all in agreement.
- Provider should count the teeth in addition to describing it.
- The carpenter's rule is an effective reminder for good provider conduct, that is:
  – Measure twice, cut once.

T: Treat the Patient

- At the beginning of the procedure, perform the second tooth count—counting aloud with the entire surgical team acknowledges the count.
- Surgical count: make sure that the assistants are engaged in the provider's actions; have them help count the teeth as a way of cross referencing (*this is the third way staff can help in preventing mistakes.*)
- Final verification (time out) should be documented in the progress notes as "Time Out performed at ___:___ hours" by the person completing the chart entry.

Clinical Settings in Which a Dentist is Most Likely to Extract the Wrong Tooth

- Third molars: extracting the molar partially covered by tissue; i.e., the second molar instead of the third molar.

- Orthodontic extractions: extracting the wrong premolar.
  - Extractions are not always conducted on the same tooth in each quadrant or arch.
- Misinterpretation or mislabeling of radiographs from an outside or even internal source.
  - If a patient presents with unmarked outside radiographs, consider taking an additional image and ensuring they are properly labeled.
- Incorrect or misunderstood referrals: clerical/paperwork missteps—often from the referral dentist's office—that the provider fails to notice.
- Surgical extractions: the tooth referred for removal is not always the tooth that appears to have the worst prognosis.
- Anatomical change in the patient's mouth between the time of referral or consultation and the date of surgery.
- Mixed dentition: proper differentiation of permanent and primary dentition is critical before initiating any dental procedure.
  - Mixed dentition may be confusing on radiographs.
  - Always double-check the referral and the teeth present in the mouth as conditions change rapidly in the mixed dentition phase.
  - When treating children, take time to show the parent/guardian exactly which tooth will be treated.

Third Molars

- Extracting a molar partially covered by tissue—often the second molar—is the most frequent clinical setting in which the wrong tooth is extracted.
- Ironically, this is probably the easiest of the wrong tooth extractions to prevent.
  - A simple tooth count will almost always prevent this surgical misadventure.
- Additional caution is required for mesially inclined second molars partially covered by soft tissue.

Wrong Premolars in Orthodontic Cases

- Dental crowding is not an automatic indication to remove all first premolars.
- Sometimes orthodontists will remove first premolars in one arch/quadrant and second premolars in another.

Radiographs

- Misinterpretation or mislabeling of radiographs by an outside or even internal source.
- It is particularly important to locate the position/orientation of impacted teeth.
  - Ensure that the laterality of the radiograph is correct.
    - Right and left sides are correct and clearly marked.

  - Supernumerary teeth (mesiodens, paramolar)
    - Facial/buccal.
    - Lingual/palatal.
- Verify the current dental condition prior to proceeding.
  - Especially important with primary teeth.
  - Primary teeth may exfoliate in the time between the consultation visit and the day of the extraction procedure.
    - Check and verify before proceeding to avoid extracting the wrong tooth.

Incorrect or Misunderstood Referrals

- There may be clerical/paperwork missteps (often from a referral dentist's office) that the provider fails to catch.
- In dentistry, the responsibility falls in the hands of the doctor holding the forceps.
- It does not matter if the errors were due to the actions of any referring or associate providers.
- If the handwriting on a referral slip is unclear, or if the tooth number on the referral slip does not correspond to a "bad tooth" or otherwise shows insufficient indication for tooth removal, do not proceed with the extraction without further confirmation from the referral office.

Surgical Extractions

- The tooth the referring dentist wants to be removed is not always the one with the poorest prognosis.
- Pay attention to previously extracted tooth sites, migration of adjacent teeth, and tipping of adjacent teeth.

Change in the Patient's Mouth

- Failing to recognize that a change has occurred in the patient's mouth between the time of referral or consultation and the date of surgery is a critical error.
- If the patient reports a dental change, or if the provider notes a dental change, consider taking a new radiograph and a new discussion with the referring dentist to re-evaluate the treatment plan prior to proceeding with a procedure.
- Always verify any uncertainties.
- Initial assumptions may not be correct.

4 Anatomy of Local Anesthesia for Dentistry*

Eric W. Baker, Julie O'Meara

General Principles of Local Anesthesia

Physiology of Peripheral Nerve Depolarization

When a nerve is inactive (not generating action potentials), there is a potential difference across its membrane which is known as the resting membrane potential (RMP) and is measured in millivolts (mV). Nerve cells have an RMP of -70 mV that is established by differences in potassium and sodium ion concentrations across the resting cell membrane—high potassium concentration intercellularly and high sodium ion concentration extracellularly. At rest, the nerve cell is relatively resistant to ion passage, but on excitation, voltage-gated sodium channels open and there is a slow influx of sodium ions into the cell. When a threshold potential is reached, depolarization occurs, and there is a fast influx of sodium ions into the cell, causing the potential across the membrane to become positive ($+40$ mV). The sodium channels quickly close again, preventing further sodium influx. At the same time, potassium channels open and there is potassium efflux from the cell. This causes repolarization of the cell membrane back to the RMP.

The depolarization of a nerve cell initiates a sequential series of depolarizations along the nerve fiber, thus propagating the impulse (action potential) along the fiber. In myelinated nerve fibers, the depolarizations "jump" from one node of Ranvier to the next (saltatory conduction). In unmyelinated fibers (which do not have nodes of Ranvier), the depolarization spreads to adjacent cells.

Mechanism of Action of Local Anesthetics

Local anesthetics block the inner (cytoplasmic) gate of sodium channels in nerve cells, preventing sodium influx and action potential initiation and propagation. Termination of action of the anesthetic at the site of injection is by diffusion of the active drug into the systemic circulation, followed by metabolism and elimination.

Duration of Anesthesia

Duration of dental local anesthesia can be defined in terms of duration of pulpal anesthesia versus the duration of soft-tissue anesthesia. Usually, dentists try to maximize the duration of pulpal anesthesia and minimize the undesirable

*Chapter reproduced from Baker EW. Anatomy for Dental Medicine, 2nd edition. Thieme ©2015; 470–487

persistence of soft-tissue anesthesia. The duration of pulpal anesthesia and the duration of soft-tissue anesthesia of some of the main local anesthetic agents following maxillary infiltration and an inferior alveolar nerve block are listed in ▶ Table 4.1.

General Injection Technique

The fingers of the supporting hand retract the soft tissue around the injection site, enabling the dentist to visualize the target area. These fingers may also be used to provide stability for the syringe and can act as reference points for some injections.

When ready to inject, the needle is inserted gently and directly, in one continuous movement, into the target area. The dentist should then aspirate to ensure that the tip of the needle does not lie within a blood vessel. Most dental syringes are "self-aspirating," meaning that if the plunger of the syringe is slightly deployed, it bounces back, aspirating (sucking) as it does so. If the syringe is not self-aspirating, aspiration is performed by drawing back slightly on the plunger. The absence of blood in the local anesthetic cartridge suggests that no vessel has been breached. If there is blood in the cartridge, the needle tip should be repositioned slightly and aspiration repeated. Following a negative aspiration result, the local anesthetic is injected slowly, exerting as little pressure as possible. Injection into the hard palate and interdental papillae are exceptions because the mucosa is tightly adherent to the supporting periosteum in these areas, necessitating that some pressure is used.

Table 4.1 Duration of anesthesia with some local anesthetic agents

Local anesthetic agent	Maxillary infiltration		Inferior alveolar nerve block	
	Duration of pulpal anesthesia (min)	Duration of soft-tissue anesthesia (min)	Duration of pulpal anesthesia (min)	Duration of soft-tissue anesthesia (min)
Lidocaine 2% with 1:100,000 epinephrine[a]	45–60	170	85	190
Articaine 4% with 1:100,000 epinephrine[a]	45–60	190	90	230
Bupivacaine 0.5% with 1:200,000 epinephrine[a]	90	340	240	440
Prilocaine 4% plain	20	105	55	190
Mepivacaine 3% plain	25	90	40	165

[a]The duration of action is prolonged when combined with epinephrine, a vasoconstrictor. A "plain" solution contains no vasoconstrictive agent.

25

Classification of Injection Techniques

Infiltration

Local anesthetic solution is deposited at the level of the tooth apices and diffuses through alveolar bone to bathe the periapical nerves.

Nerve Blocks

Local anesthetic solution is deposited around the main nerve trunk and therefore anesthetizes all of the branches distal to it.

Overview of Nerves Anesthetized

Injections given within the oral cavity anesthetize a branch or branches of either the maxillary or mandibular division of the trigeminal nerve (CN V_2 or CN V_3, respectively) on the same side as the injection (▶ Fig. 4.1 and ▶ Fig. 4.2).

Failure of Anesthesia

Patient Variation

A typical dose of local anesthetic profoundly anesthetizes some patients but may not sufficiently anesthetize others. The dentist must try to ascertain

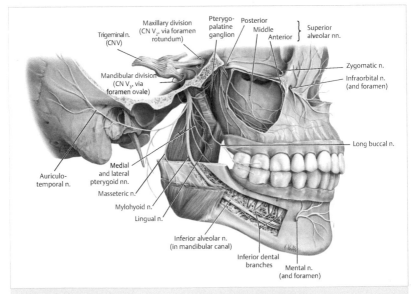

Fig. 4.1 Trigeminal nerve in the oral cavity. Right lateral view. (From Schuenke M, Schulte E, Schumacher U. THIEME Atlas of Anatomy. Head, Neck, and Neuroanatomy. Illustrations by Voll M and Wesker K. Second Edition. New York: Thieme Medical Publishers; 2016).

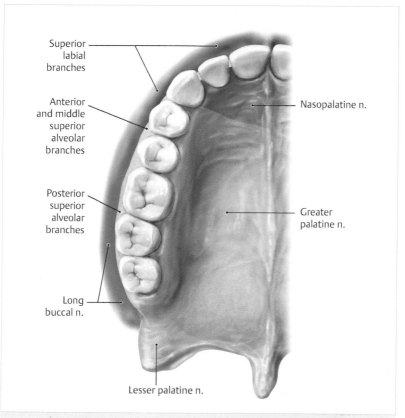

Fig. 4.2 Innervation of the hard palate. Inferior view. (From Baker EW. Anatomy for Dental Medicine. Illustrations by Voll M and Wesker K. Second Edition. New York: Thieme Medical Publishers; 2015).

whether failure is due to patient variation or improper injection technique. If due to the former, then more local anesthetic may be given to achieve adequate anesthesia. Likewise, differences occur between patients in the duration of action of anesthetics. The best way to mitigate these differences is to begin treatment as soon as anesthesia is achieved, i.e., ~ 2 minutes after injection for an infiltration and ~ 5 minutes after injection for a block.

Acute Pulpitis or Apical Abscess

Acute pulpitis (pulpal inflammation) results in a hyperemic tooth (a tooth in which the pulpal blood vessels dilate causing a painful increase in pressure) that is difficult to adequately anesthetize. The pus of an apical abscess can prevent proper diffusion of the local anesthetic solution to the periapical nerves and vessels.

Intravascular Injection

If all or part of an injection of local anesthetic is deposited intravascularly then there may be little or no anesthesia achieved.

Injection into Muscles or Their Fascia

If the local anesthetic is deposited in a muscle or its fascia instead of the bone near the teeth apices, then the distance the anesthetic has to diffuse to reach the apical nerves and vessels is increased, resulting in reduced anesthesia. Injection into a muscle can also produce trismus (restricted mouth opening).

Complications and Their Treatment

Fainting

This is the most common systemic complication and is likely attributed to anxiety over the procedure. It can be minimized by administering local anesthetic with the patient in supine position. If fainting does occur, place the patient in a supine position, and recovery will occur rapidly.

Allergic Reactions

Allergy to local anesthetic is uncommon but possible. It may be due to allergy to the drug, allergy to the additives for compounding the drug, or latex allergy to the rubber bung located at one end of a local anesthetic cartridge. Allergy manifests as facial flushing, swelling, rash, itching, and wheezing. The patient should be sent for allergy testing to determine the precise cause. For minor allergic reactions, provide reassurance and antihistamines if necessary. For severe (anaphylactic) reactions, urgently call for an ambulance, place the patient in a supine position, and give emergency medication as needed (e.g., intramuscular epinephrine, intravenous hydrocortisone, and oxygen by mask).

Cardiovascular Collapse

Cardiovascular collapse may be precipitated by, or exacerbated by stress, excessive amounts of local anesthetic, and improper aspiration, leading to deposition of local anesthetic in a blood vessel. Epinephrine in the local anesthetic can act directly on the heart, which, if previously diseased, can cause arrhythmias.

If this occurs, urgently call for an ambulance, place the patient in a supine position, and maintain airway and circulation.

Hematomas

Small hematomas are of little consequence, but larger hematomas can compromise the airway. No treatment is needed for small hematomas; whereas large hematomas due to arterial bleeding, if they are not self-limiting, may require ligation of the vessel.

Trismus

Trismus is the inability to open the mouth normally. It usually occurs after an inferior alveolar nerve block that is given too low, resulting in hematoma formation in the medial pterygoid. This may be accompanied by infection. Treatment includes reassurance, antibiotics, and encouragement to progressively try to open the mouth.

Facial Paralysis

Facial paralysis (or palsy) may occur following an improperly placed inferior alveolar nerve block. If the needle is directed too far posteriorly, the tip may enter the superficial layer of deep cervical fascia that surrounds the parotid gland. Thus the local anesthetic is able to penetrate the gland and anesthetize the five branches of the facial nerve that are embedded within it. This is manifested by the patient's inability to frown or blink and drooping of the mouth on the affected side. The facial paralysis is transient, normally lasting for ~ 1 hour.

Treatment includes reassurance and a protective eye covering until the blink reflex returns.

Maxillary Anesthesia

Maxillary Incisors and Canines

Anatomy

The incisors and canines and their associated periodontal ligaments, buccal gingiva, mucosa, and supporting bone are innervated by the anterior superior alveolar nerves which branch off the infraorbital nerve just before it emerges from the infraorbital foramen (▶ Table 4.2). These nerves anastomose over the midline. The palatal gingiva, mucosa, and supporting bone are innervated by the nasopalatine nerve, which emerges through the incisive foramen.

The medial spread of local anesthetic may be hindered by the labial frenulum that anchors the lip to the attached gingiva in the midline.

The maxillary bone has a thin, porous lamina (layer) easily penetrated by an infiltration of local anesthetic solution.

Table 4.2 Anesthesia of maxillary incisors and canine

Areas anesthetized[a] (see ▶ Fig. 4.3c and ▶ Fig. 4.3d)	Nerve (▶ Fig. 4.3b)
Maxillary central, lateral incisor[a] and canine[b] and their associated periodontal ligaments, buccal gingiva, mucosa, and supporting bone	Anterior superior alveolar nerve
Lateral aspect of the nose	External nasal branch fibers of the infraorbital nerve
Upper lip	Superior labial branch fibers of the infraorbital nerve

[a]This applies when the injection is placed superior to the maxillary lateral incisor.
[b]The root of the canine is longer and the apical part of the root is often distally oriented; therefore, the maxillary right canine may not be sufficiently anesthetized for cavity preparation from this injection alone.

Injection Technique

- Insert the needle in the mucobuccal fold immediately superior to the crown of the tooth being anesthetized and pass it axially toward the apex of the tooth (▶ Fig. 4.3a, b). The needle should be in close proximity to the bone to ensure that the local anesthetic solution has minimal diffusion distance before it bathes the periapical nerves and vessels.
- Following a negative aspiration result, slowly inject 1.0 to 1.8 mL of local anesthetic.
- For central incisors, the injection is best placed distally due to the close proximity of the anterior nasal spine.

Clinical Considerations

- A mucobuccal fold infiltration is sufficient for cavity preparation and pulpal procedures.
- Extractions will require supplementary anesthesia of the palatal gingiva, mucosa, and supporting bone, either by local infiltration of the palate or by a nasopalatine block.
- It is a painful injection.

Infraorbital Nerve Block

Anatomy

The infraorbital nerve is a continuation of the maxillary nerve as it enters the infraorbital canal. The anterior superior alveolar nerve and middle superior alveolar nerve (when present) branch from this nerve just before it exits the infraorbital canal and are, therefore, also anesthetized by diffusion of local anesthetic from the injection site (▶ Table 4.3).

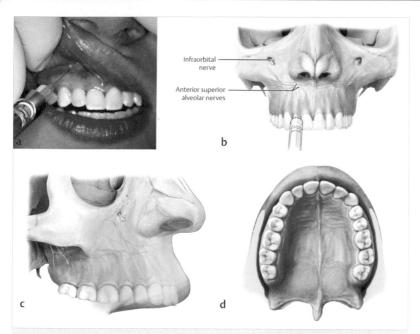

Fig. 4.3 Infiltration of the maxillary lateral incisor. (**a**) Injection technique. (**b**) Nerves anesthetized, anterior view. (**c**) Areas anesthetized, right lateral view. (**d**) Areas anesthetized, inferior view. Note the lips roughly extend to the first premolar region on each side; the cheeks are colored gray. (From Baker EW. Anatomy for Dental Medicine. Illustrations by Voll M and Wesker K. Second Edition. New York: Thieme Medical Publishers; 2015).

Table 4.3 Anesthesia following an infraorbital nerve block

Areas anesthetized (▶ Fig. 4.4c and ▶ Fig. 4.4d)	Nerve (▶ Fig. 4.4b)
Incisors and canine and their associated periodontal ligament, buccal gingiva, mucosa, and supporting bone	Anterior superior alveolar nerve
Premolars and possibly the mesiobuccal cusp of the first molar and their associated periodontal ligament, buccal gingiva, mucosa, and supporting bone	Middle superior alveolar nerve or fibers from the superior dental plexus
Lateral aspect of the nose	External nasal branches of the infraorbital nerve
Lower eyelid	Inferior palpebral branches of the infraorbital nerve
Upper lip and mucosa	Superior labial branches of the infraorbital nerve

Injection Technique

- Palpate the center of the inferior margin of the orbit with the index finger of the supporting hand. At a point ~ 1 cm below the orbital margin, the infraorbital foramen can be palpated. Hold the index finger at that point, while retracting the upper lip with the thumb of the supporting hand. Insert the needle at the mucobuccal fold immediately superior to the first maxillary premolar, parallel to the long axis of the tooth, toward the tip of the index finger (▶ Fig. 4.4a, b).
- Following a negative aspiration result, slowly inject ~ 1 mL of local anesthetic.

Clinical Considerations

- To avoid having to give more than one injection, an infraorbital block may be used to anesthetize multiple teeth for cavity preparation or pulpal procedures. It may also be used when infiltration has failed to achieve

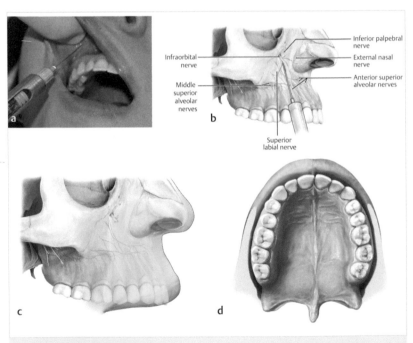

Fig. 4.4 Infraorbital nerve block. (a) Injection technique. (b) Nerves anesthetized, right lateral view. (c) Areas anesthetized, right lateral view. (d) Areas anesthetized, inferior view. (From Baker EW. Anatomy for Dental Medicine. Illustrations by Voll M and Wesker K. Second Edition. New York: Thieme Medical Publishers; 2015).

pulpal anesthesia or is contraindicated (e.g., infiltration would require an injection into an infected area).

- Extractions of any of the teeth anesthetized by an infraorbital block will require supplementary anesthesia of the palatal gingiva by a nasopalatine or greater palatine block or by local infiltration of the palate.
- Hematoma is rare with this injection, but there is potential for iatrogenic (accidental, clinician-induced) damage to the patient's eye.
- To obtain complete anesthesia of the central incisor on the same side as the injection, it may be necessary to block anastomosing fibers from the anterior superior alveolar nerve on the contralateral side of the midline. This is achieved by placing a supplemental 0.5 mL of local anesthetic in the contralateral buccal fold just distal to the central incisor.

Maxillary Premolars

Anatomy

The premolar area is innervated by the superior dental plexus, which is formed by convergent branches from the posterior superior alveolar nerve and the anterior superior alveolar nerve. Sometimes there is a middle superior alveolar nerve that, when present, innervates the premolars, their periodontal ligaments, buccal gingiva, and supporting bone, and often the mesiobuccal root of the first molar (▶ Table 4.4). The palatal gingiva, mucosa, and supporting bone adjacent to the premolars is mainly innervated by the greater palatine nerve, but the area of the first premolar may also be innervated by fibers of the nasopalatine nerve.

Diffusion of local anesthetic deposited in the mucobuccal fold is especially good in this area because the bone lamina is thin and the apices of the premolars lie very close to the lamina. Consequently, small volumes of local anesthetic are required, and the palatal roots of the premolars are almost always anesthetized by this one injection.

Table 4.4 Anesthesia of maxillary premolars

Area anesthetized[a] (▶ Fig. 4.5c and ▶ Fig. 4.5d)	Nerve (▶ Fig. 4.5b)
Both maxillary premolars[a] and their associated periodontal ligaments, buccal gingiva, mucosa, and supporting bone	Middle superior alveolar nerve or branches of the superior dental plexus
Canine and the mesiobuccal cusp of the first molar[b] and their associated periodontal ligaments, buccal gingiva, mucosa, and supporting bone	

[a]This applies when the injection is placed between the premolars.
[b]These teeth, soft tissues, and bone may also be anesthetized to a lesser extent.

Injection Technique

The same infiltration technique is used in this case as for the incisors and canines. Deposit 1.0 to 1.5 mL of local anesthetic solution around the apex of the premolars (► Fig. 4.5**a, b**).

Clinical Considerations

- A mucobuccal fold infiltration is sufficient for cavity preparation and pulpal procedures.
- Extractions will require supplementary anesthesia of the palatal gingiva, mucosa, and supporting bone, usually by one local infiltration injection of the palate between the premolars.

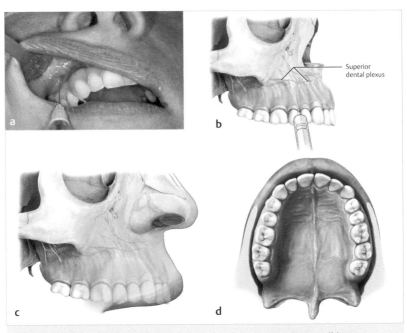

Fig. 4.5 Infiltration of the maxillary premolars. (**a**) Injection technique. (**b**) Nerves anesthetized, right lateral view. (**c**) Areas anesthetized, right lateral view. (**d**) Areas anesthetized, inferior view. ([a]: From Daubländer M in van Aken H, Wulf H: Lokalanästhesie, Regionalanästhesie, Regionale Schmerztherapie. Third Edition. Stuttgart: Thieme; 2010; [b-d]: From Baker EW. Anatomy for Dental Medicine. Illustrations by Voll M and Wesker K. Second Edition. New York: Thieme Medical Publishers; 2015).

Maxillary Molars

Anatomy

The molar region of the maxilla is innervated by the posterior superior alveolar nerve, which branches from the infraorbital nerve before it enters the infraorbital canal. These branches enter foramina on the infratemporal surface of the maxilla, where they enter to innervate the maxillary molars and their associated periodontal ligaments, buccal gingiva, mucosa, and supporting bone (▶ Table 4.5). The distance between the mucobuccal fold and the apices of the maxillary molars varies from patient to patient. This distance may be increased by the lower margin of the zygomatic arch or when the maxillary sinus extends down between the buccal and palatal roots. This can lead to failure of a buccal infiltration injection.

Injection Technique

- The same infiltration technique as for incisors and canines is used. Introduce the needle to the mucobuccal fold slightly mesially to the maxillary first molar (▶ Fig. 4.6a, b). A second injection may be given in the mucobuccal fold at the distal aspect of the maxillary first molar to ensure the tooth is adequately anesthetized.
- Following a negative aspiration result, slowly inject 1.0 to 1.7 mL of local anesthetic.

Clinical Considerations

- A mucobuccal fold infiltration injection is usually sufficient for cavity preparation and pulpal procedures. Rarely, it may be necessary to perform a palatal injection to achieve complete anesthesia of the palatal root.
- Extractions will require supplementary anesthesia of the palatal gingiva, mucosa, and supporting bone by greater palatine block or by local infiltration.

Table 4.5 Anesthesia of maxillary molars

Area anesthetized[a] (▶ Fig. 4.6c and ▶ Fig. 4.6d)	Nerve (▶ Fig. 4.6b)
Mesiobuccal cusp of the first molar	Middle superior alveolar nerve (if present)
First and second molar[a] and their associated periodontal ligaments, buccal gingiva, mucosa, and supporting bone	Posterior superior alveolar nerve
Lateral aspect of the lip (may be very slight or absent)	Superior labial branches of the infraorbital nerve

[a]This applies when injection is placed mesially and distally to the first molar.

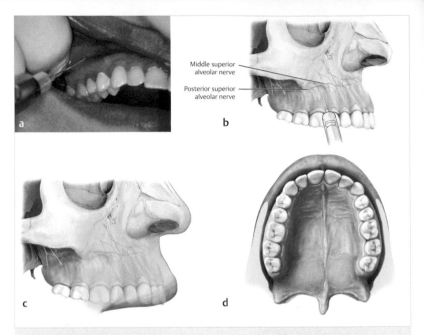

Fig. 4.6 Infiltration of the maxillary molars. (**a**) Injection technique. (**b**) Nerves anesthetized, right lateral view. (**c**) Areas anesthetized, right lateral view. (**d**) Areas anesthetized, inferior view. (From Baker EW. Anatomy for Dental Medicine. Illustrations by Voll M and Wesker K. Second Edition. New York: Thieme Medical Publishers; 2015).

- For infiltration injections of the maxillary third molars, the patient should not be asked to open too widely; otherwise, the coronoid process of the mandible is moved anteriorly and can cover the injection site.

Posterior Superior Alveolar Nerve Block

Anatomy

The posterior superior alveolar nerve is located in the infratemporal fossa and lies in close proximity to the pterygoid plexus of veins (▶ Table 4.6).

Injection Technique

- Instruct the patient to open his or her mouth and swing the mandible toward the same side to allow better visualization of the injection site and more room to maneuver.

- Insert the needle into the mucobuccal fold just superior to the maxillary second molar, between the medial border of the ramus of the mandible and the maxillary tuberosity. Then advance the needle inward, backward, and upward 1.5 to 2.0 cm (▶ Fig. 4.7a, b).
- Following a negative aspiration result, slowly deposit 1.0 to 1.7 mL of local anesthetic.

Table 4.6 Anesthesia following a posterior superior alveolar nerve block

Areas anesthetized[a] (▶ Fig. 4.7c and ▶ Fig. 4.7d)	Nerve (▶ Fig. 4.7b)
Maxillary first,[a] second, and third molars and their associated periodontal ligaments, buccal gingiva, mucosa, and supporting bone	Posterior superior alveolar nerve

[a]The mesiobuccal root of the first molar may not be anesthetized and may, therefore, require supplemental buccal infiltration anesthesia mesial to the first molar (to anesthetize the middle superior alveolar nerve).

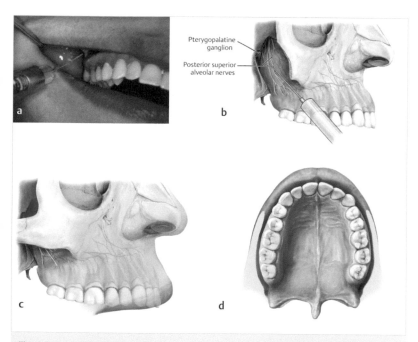

Fig. 4.7 Posterior superior alveolar nerve block. (**a**) Injection technique. (**b**) Nerves anesthetized, right lateral view. (**c**) Areas anesthetized, right lateral view. (**d**) Areas anesthetized, inferior view. (From Baker EW. Anatomy for Dental Medicine. Illustrations by Voll M and Wesker K. Second Edition. New York: Thieme Medical Publishers; 2015).

Clinical Considerations

- This injection is sufficient for cavity preparation and pulpal procedures on all of the maxillary molars.
- Extractions will require supplementary anesthesia of the palatal gingiva, mucosa, and supporting bone by a greater palatine nerve block or by local infiltration.

Notes

There is a significant risk of hematoma by introduction of the needle into the pterygoid plexus. Short needles and careful aspiration reduce this risk.

Maxillary Division Block

Anatomy

The maxillary division block is an advanced local anesthetic technique. It uses the greater palatine canal to reach the pterygopalatine fossa and, therefore, enables the dentist to anesthetize all branches of the maxillary nerve (▶ Table 4.7). The canal is usually vertical, thus aiding this procedure.

Injection Technique

- Locate the greater palatine foramen with a cotton swab applicator, which can be felt to sink slightly into the foramen. Inject a small amount of anesthetic. This lessens patient's discomfort for the next part of the procedure.
- Insert the needle into the greater palatine foramen ~ 28 to 30 mm. The needle tip should now be located in the pterygopalatine fossa (▶ Fig. 4.8a, b).
- Following a negative aspiration result, slowly inject 1 to 2 mL of local anesthetic.

Table 4.7 Anesthesia following a maxillary division block

Areas anesthetized (▶ Fig. 4.8c and ▶ Fig. 4.8d)	Nerve (▶ Fig. 4.8b)
All maxillary teeth and their associated periodontal ligaments, buccal gingiva, mucosa, and supporting bone	Anterior, middle (if present), and posterior superior alveolar nerves
All palatal gingival, mucosa, and supporting bone	Nasopalatine nerve (anterior one-third) and greater palatine nerve (posterior two-thirds)
Lateral aspect of the nose	External nasal branches of the infraorbital nerve
Lower eyelid	Inferior palpebral branches of the infraorbital nerve
Upper lip	Superior labial branches of the infraorbital nerve

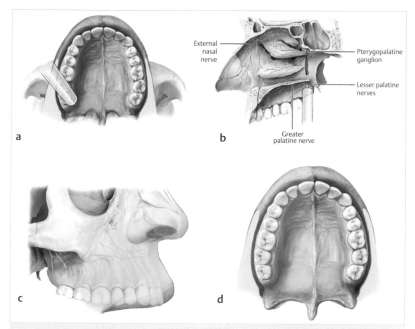

Fig. 4.8 Maxillary division block. (**a**) Injection technique, inferior view. (**b**) Nerves anesthetized, left lateral view of the right lateral nasal wall with the pterygopalatine ganglion exposed. (**c**) Areas anesthetized, right lateral view. (**d**) Areas anesthetized, inferior view. (From Baker EW. Anatomy for Dental Medicine. Illustrations by Voll M and Wesker K. Second Edition. New York: Thieme Medical Publishers; 2015).

Clinical Considerations

- This injection is useful when extensive restorative dentistry and surgical procedures are needed.
- The needle should never be forced into the greater palatine foramen to avoid fracture of the wall of the greater palatine canal.
- If the needle is placed too far superiorly, the anesthetic can be deposited in the eye, affecting vision.
- Hematoma formation may occur due to rupture of the vessels that also run in the greater palatine canal.

Nasopalatine Nerve Block

Anatomy

The nasopalatine nerve is a branch of the maxillary nerve that passes through the pterygopalatine ganglion (▶ Table 4.8). It enters the nasal cavity through

Table 4.8 Anesthesia following a nasopalatine nerve block

Area anesthetized (▶ Fig. 4.9c)	Nerve (▶ Fig. 4.9b)
The maxillary gingiva, mucosa, and supporting bone from the right maxillary canine to the left maxillary canine	Nasopalatine nerve

the sphenopalatine foramen, passes across the roof of the nasal cavity, then runs obliquely downward and forward in the nasal septum between the supporting bone and mucous membrane. It descends farther through the incisive canal and emerges into the anterior hard palate through the incisive foramen. Branches of the nasopalatine nerve anastomose with branches of the contralateral nasopalatine nerve and with the greater palatine nerve. Because the right and left nasopalatine nerves exit the incisive foramen in close proximity, one injection anesthetizes both sides of the anterior one-third of the hard palate.

Injection Technique

- Using a cotton swab applicator, apply pressure close to the injection site to reduce the perception of pain. Insert the needle into the palatal mucosa lateral to the incisive papilla until bone is contacted (▶ Fig. 4.9**a, b**).
- After withdrawing the needle slightly and following a negative aspiration result, inject a very small volume of local anesthetic under minimal pressure. The tissue will be seen to blanch due to the vasoconstrictor in the local anesthetic solution.

Clinical Considerations

- This injection is used to supplement buccal infiltration injections for extraction of any of the maxillary anterior teeth.
- This injection is widely perceived to be the most painful variety of dental injection. It is particularly painful because the mucosa of the hard palate is tightly bound to the periosteum of the palate, allowing little space for the diffusion of local anesthetic.

Greater Palatine Nerve Block

Anatomy

The greater palatine nerve is a branch of the maxillary nerve that passes through the greater palatine ganglion (▶ Table 4.9). It runs from the pterygopalatine fossa, down through the greater palatine canal, and through the greater palatine foramen to reach the hard palate. It then runs forward in a groove to a point just distal to the canine tooth.

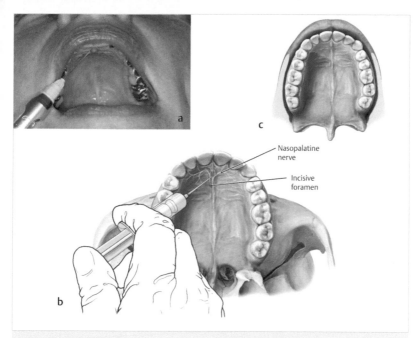

Fig. 4.9 Nasopalatine nerve block. (**a**) Injection technique, inferior view. (**b**) Nerves anesthetized, inferior view. (**c**) Areas anesthetized, inferior view. ([a]: From Daubländer M in van Aken H, Wulf H: Lokalanästhesie, Regionalanästhesie, Regionale Schmerztherapie. Third Edition. Stuttgart: Thieme; 2010; [b,c]: From Baker EW. Anatomy for Dental Medicine. Illustrations by Voll M and Wesker K. Second Edition. New York: Thieme Medical Publishers; 2015).

Table 4.9 Anesthesia following a greater palatine nerve block

Area anesthetized (▶ Fig. 4.10c)	Nerve (▶ Fig. 4.10b)
The maxillary gingiva, mucosa, and supporting bone from the maxillary first premolar to the posterior hard palate to the midline of the hard palate	Greater palatine nerve

Injection Technique

- The greater palatine foramen lies ~ 0.5 to 1.0 cm mesial to the margin of the gingiva at the distal border of the maxillary second molar (▶ Fig. 4.10a, b). It should be located by using a cotton swab applicator, as it can be felt to sink slightly into the foramen. With the cotton swab applicator, apply pressure close to the injection site to reduce the perception of pain. Insert the needle until it contacts bone. Withdraw it slightly, then aspirate.
- Following a negative aspiration result, slowly inject around 0.1 mL of local anesthetic.

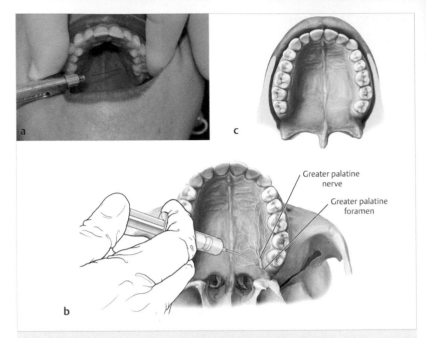

Fig. 4.10 Greater palatine nerve block. (a) Injection technique, inferior view. (b) Nerves anesthetized, inferior view. (c) Areas anesthetized, inferior view. (From Baker EW. Anatomy for Dental Medicine. Illustrations by Voll M and Wesker K. Second Edition. New York: Thieme Medical Publishers; 2015).

Clinical Considerations

- This injection is used to anesthetize palatal tissues for multiple extractions involving the maxillary premolars and molars on one side. It may also be useful for mucogingival surgical procedures.
- Bone contact prior to injection is necessary to ensure that the needle is not in the soft palate.
- The palate in the region of the greater palatine foramen is tightly bound to the supporting bone but less so than at the incisive foramen. Therefore, although still painful, this injection is less so than for the nasopalatine nerve block.

Supplementary Infiltration of the Palate

Anatomy

Supplementary infiltration of the palate may anesthetize fibers of the nasopalatine nerve and/or greater palatine nerve (depending on the site of the injection; ▶ Table 4.10).

Injection Technique

- Using a cotton swab applicator, apply pressure close to the injection site to reduce the perception of pain. Insert the needle into the palatal mucosa ~ 1 cm from the neck of the tooth to be anesthetized, until bone is contacted.
- Withdraw the needle slightly and aspirate.
- Following a negative aspiration result, inject ~ 0.1 mL of local anesthetic. The mucosa will be seen to blanch due to the vasoconstrictor in the local anesthetic.

Clinical Considerations

- This injection is used to supplement buccal infiltration, infraorbital, or posterior superior alveolar nerve blocks for extractions of the maxillary teeth. It is more commonly performed than a nasopalatine or greater palatine nerve block.
- The injection is painful.

Mandibular Anesthesia

Mandibular Incisors and Canines

Anatomy

The incisors and canines are innervated by the incisive nerve, a terminal branch of the inferior alveolar nerve (▶ Table 4.11). Its course lies within bone, but it may be anesthetized by infiltration because the bone lamina in this area of the mandible is thin and porous. As the bone around the canine teeth in adults may be denser, infiltration anesthesia may fail. In this case, a mental nerve block or inferior alveolar nerve block can be used to ensure sufficient anesthesia of a canine tooth.

Table 4.10 Supplementary infiltration of the palate

Areas anesthetized	Nerve
Palatal gingiva, mucosa, and supporting bone in the vicinity of the injection site	Fibers of the nasopalatine nerve and/or greater palatine nerve

Table 4.11 Anesthesia of mandibular incisors and canine

Areas anesthetized[a] (▶ Fig. 4.11c)	Nerve (▶ Fig. 4.11b)
Mandibular central and lateral incisors and canine (to a lesser extent)[a]	Incisive nerve
Periodontal ligaments, buccal gingiva, mucosa, and supporting bone associated with the incisors	Mental nerve
Lower lip	
Chin	

[a]This applies when the injection is placed at the mandibular lateral incisor.

43

The buccal soft tissues are innervated by the mental nerve, while the lingual gingiva and supporting bone are supplied by the sublingual nerve (a branch of the lingual nerve).

Injection Technique

The same infiltration technique is used as for the maxillary incisors and canines. Deposit around 1 mL of local anesthetic around the apices of the teeth (▶ Fig. 4.11a, b; ▶ Table 4.11).

Clinical Considerations

- A mucobuccal fold injection is sufficient for cavity preparation and pulpal procedures of the mandibular incisors.
- Extractions require supplemental anesthesia of the lingual gingiva, mucosa, and supporting bone by sublingual infiltration.

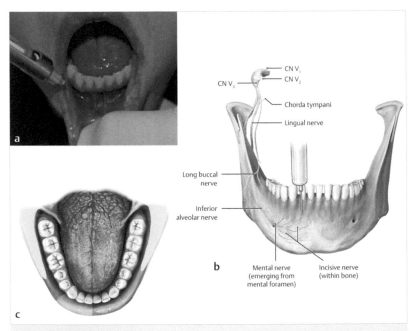

Fig. 4.11 Infiltration of the mandibular incisors. (**a**) Injection technique, anterior view. (**b**) Nerves anesthetized, anterior view. (**c**) Areas anesthetized, superior view. (From Baker EW. Anatomy for Dental Medicine. Illustrations by Voll M and Wesker K. Second Edition. New York: Thieme Medical Publishers; 2015).

Mental Nerve Block

Anatomy

The mandibular first premolar is innervated by the mental nerve in the mandibular canal (▶ Table 4.12). The mandibular second premolar is mainly innervated by the inferior alveolar nerve. The periodontal ligaments, buccal gingiva, mucosa, and supporting bone in the premolar area are innervated by the mental nerve, while the lingual gingiva is supplied by the sublingual nerve. The mental foramen lies between and inferior to the apices of the mandibular premolar teeth.

The thick, compact bone in the mandibular premolar region does not normally allow anesthesia of these teeth to be achieved by infiltration anesthesia; therefore, a mental nerve block or inferior alveolar nerve block is used. The exception to this is if articaine is used; in that case, infiltration anesthesia is effective (articaine can achieve anesthesia of all mandibular teeth with the exception of the second and third molars).

The anatomic direction of the canal that allows passage of the mental nerve is medial → anterior → caudal. The needle should not be oriented in this direction to prevent damage to the mental nerve and vessels within the canal.

Injection Technique

- Locate the mental foramen by palpation or by referring to a radiograph.
- Insert the needle into the mucobuccal fold between the first and second mandibular premolar.
- Advance the needle until it is at the level of the mental foramen (▶ Fig. 4.12**a, b**).

Table 4.12 Anesthesia following a mental nerve block

Areas anesthetized[a] (▶ Fig. 4.12c)	Nerve (▶ Fig. 4.12b)
Mandibular first premolar	Mental nerve
Mandibular second premolar[a]	Inferior alveolar nerve and perhaps some fibers from the mental nerve
Canine, lateral, and central incisor	Incisive nerve[b]
All periodontal ligaments, buccal gingiva, mucosa, and supporting bone from the second premolar to the central incisor	Mental nerve
Lower lip and chin	Mental nerve

[a]Unreliably anesthetized, as sufficient anesthetic has to diffuse through the mental foramen and spread distally to anesthetize fibers of the inferior alveolar nerve, which innervates this tooth.
[b]The incisive nerve is incidentally anesthetized by diffusion of local anesthetic during this block.

45

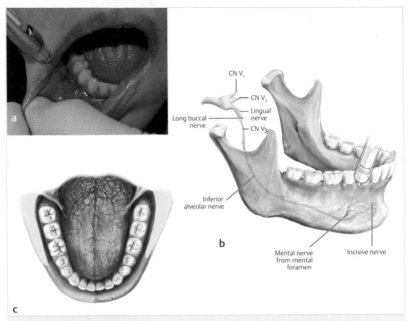

Fig. 4.12 Mental nerve block. (**a**) Injection technique. (**b**) Nerves anesthetized, right lateral view. (**c**) Areas anesthetized, superior view. (From Baker EW. Anatomy for Dental Medicine. Illustrations by Voll M and Wesker K. Second Edition. New York: Thieme Medical Publishers; 2015).

- Following a negative aspiration result, slowly inject 1.0 to 1.5 mL of local anesthetic.

Clinical Considerations

- This injection is sufficient for cavity preparation and pulpal procedures on the mandibular first premolar. Cavity preparation may be performed on the mandibular second premolar if anesthesia permits, but pulpal procedures and extensive cavity preparations are likely to require an inferior alveolar nerve block to be performed for adequate anesthesia.
- For extractions of the mandibular first premolar, a supplementary sublingual nerve infiltration is required. For extractions of the mandibular second premolar, an inferior alveolar nerve block is performed during which the lingual nerve is concurrently blocked.

Inferior Alveolar Nerve Block

Anatomy

All mandibular teeth are innervated by the inferior alveolar nerve (and its branches) that runs in the mandibular canal (▶ Table 4.13).

The thick, compact bone in the mandibular molar region often does not allow for infiltration anesthesia. Therefore, anesthesia of the mandibular molars requires blockade of the inferior alveolar nerve before it enters the mandibular canal. However, an infiltration injection of articaine has been shown to be effective in anesthetizing all mandibular teeth except the second and third molars.

Injection Technique

- Instruct the patient to open the mouth widely to ensure good visualization of the anatomic landmarks.
- Palpate the coronoid notch of the mandible with the thumb of the supporting hand.
- The deepest part of the coronoid notch (about halfway up the thumb) generally corresponds to the level of the mandibular foramen.
- Move the thumb medially to palpate the internal oblique ridge and then the pterygomandibular space, lateral to the pterygomandibular raphe. The index and middle fingers lie at the ramus and angle of the mandible to support the mandible.
- Direct the needle from the contralateral premolar area into the pterygomandibular space at the level of the mandibular foramen, while keeping the needle parallel to the occlusal plane of the mandibular teeth on the injection side.
- Insert the needle 20 to 25 mm until bone is contacted (▶ Fig. 4.13**a**, **b**).
- Withdraw the needle slightly, then aspirate.

Table 4.13 Anesthesia following an inferior alveolar nerve block

Areas anesthetized[a] (▶ Fig. 4.13c and ▶ Fig. 4.13d)	Nerve (▶ Fig. 4.13b)
All mandibular teeth	Inferior alveolar nerve
All buccal gingiva, mucosa, and supporting bone from the second premolar to the central incisor	Mental nerve
Lower lip and chin	Mental nerve
All lingual gingiva, mucosa, and supporting bone	Lingual nerve (molar region) and its sublingual branch (premolar region to midline)
Anterior two-thirds of the tongue	Lingual nerve

[a]On the same side as the injection.

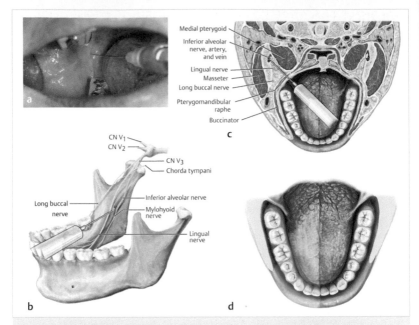

Fig. 4.13 Inferior alveolar nerve block. (**a**) Injection technique. (**b**) Nerves anesthetized, left lateral view. (**c**) Transverse section just above the occlusal plane of the mandibular teeth, superior view. (**d**) Areas anesthetized, superior view. ([**a**]: From Daubländer M in van Aken H, Wulf H: Lokalanästhesie, Regionalanästhesie, Regionale Schmerztherapie. Third Edition. Stuttgart: Thieme; 2010; [**b-d**]: From Baker EW. Anatomy for Dental Medicine. Illustrations by Voll M and Wesker K. Second Edition. New York: Thieme Medical Publishers; 2015).

- Following a negative aspiration result, slowly inject ~ 1.5 mL of local anesthetic into the pterygomandibular space.
- The lingual nerve is concurrently blocked by withdrawing the needle about halfway (corresponding to the approximate level of the temporal crest), aspirating, and slowly injecting the remaining 0.5 mL of local anesthetic if aspiration is negative.

Clinical Considerations

- This injection is sufficient for cavity preparations, pulpal procedures, and surgical procedures involving the lingual aspect of the mandibular teeth.
- Extractions of the mandibular molars require supplemental anesthesia of the long buccal nerve.
- The patient may describe an "electric shock" if the tip of the needle directly touches the inferior alveolar nerve. In this case, the needle should be withdrawn slightly, as the nerve may be damaged by intraneural injection, and the symptoms are often persistent.

- The mandibular foramen is not at the same level in all patients; therefore, this technique has to be modified accordingly. In children, it is located closer to the posterior border of the mandible until more bone is produced. In edentulous patients, alveolar bone resorption has occurred, making the deepest part of the coronoid notch lower than normal. To avoid making the block too low, direct the needle higher than the deepest part of the coronoid notch.
- In class II malocclusion, when the mandible is hypoplastic (underdeveloped), the mandibular foramen may be located more inferior than normal.
- In class III malocclusion, when the mandible is hyperplastic (overdeveloped) the mandibular foramen may be located more superior than normal.
- The medial pterygoid muscle is stretched and tense if the mouth is opened widely and may hinder proper placement of the needle. This can be overcome by slightly reducing the mouth opening after the initial insertion of the needle.
- If the needle is angled too far mesially, the bone of the temporal crest is contacted almost immediately, and the needle should be repositioned laterally. If the needle is inserted too far posteriorly, then deposition of the local anesthetic solution may be made in the medial pterygoid muscle, causing postoperative muscle pain and trismus (muscle spasm). If the needle continues farther posteriorly, then it may penetrate the capsule of the parotid gland. If local anesthetic is deposited within the capsule, it causes a transient facial paralysis (Bell's palsy). Ensuring that the needle contacts bone at the appropriate depth ensures proper placement and mitigates the likelihood of any complications.

Gow—Gates Block

Anatomy

This block is a variation of the inferior alveolar nerve block. The aim is to anesthetize the inferior alveolar nerve at the level of the mandibular condyle, but additional branches of CN V_3 are also anesthetized by at injection given at this level (▶ Table 4.14).

Injection Technique

- Instruct the patient to open the mouth as wide as possible.
- Direct the needle from the contralateral premolars and insert the needle high into the mucosa at the level of the maxillary second molar, just distal to the mesiolingual cusp (▶ Fig. 4.14**a, b**).
- Use the intertragic notch of the ear as an extraoral landmark to help reach the neck of the mandibular condyle.
- When contact with the neck of the condyle is made, withdraw the needle slightly and aspirate.

Table 4.14 Anesthesia following a Gow—Gates block

Area anesthetized[a] (▶ Fig. 4.14c)	Nerve (▶ Fig. 4.14b)
All mandibular teeth	Inferior alveolar nerve
All periodontal ligaments, buccal gingiva, mucosa, and supporting alveolar bone from the second premolar to the third molar	Long buccal nerve
All periodontal ligaments, buccal gingiva, mucosa, and supporting alveolar bone from the second premolar to the central incisor	Mental nerve
All lingual gingiva, supporting bone, and the mucosa of the floor of the mouth	Lingual nerve (molar region) and its sublingual branch (premolar to midline)
Anterior two-thirds of the tongue	Lingual nerve
Lower lip	Mental nerve
Skin in the temple region and the skin anterior to the ear	Auriculotemporal nerve
Posterior part of the cheek	Long buccal nerve

[a]On the same side as the injection.

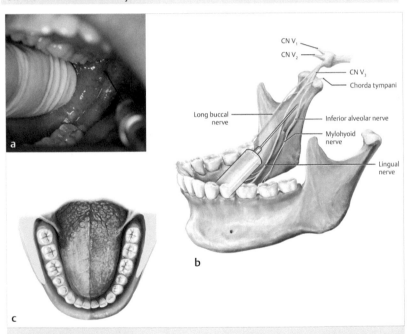

Fig. 4.14 Gow—Gates block. (**a**) Injection technique. (**b**) Nerves anesthetized, left lateral view. (**c**) Areas anesthetized, superior view. (From Baker EW. Anatomy for Dental Medicine. Illustrations by Voll M and Wesker K. Second Edition. New York: Thieme Medical Publishers; 2015).

- Following a negative aspiration result, slowly inject 1.0 to 1.7 mL of local anesthetic.

Clinical Considerations

- This injection is useful for multiple procedures on mandibular teeth and buccal soft tissue.
- The rate of failure is lower and there are fewer aspiration issues than with the traditional inferior alveolar nerve block.

Akinosi Block

Anatomy

The Akinosi block is an alternative, closed-mouth method of performing an inferior alveolar nerve block (▶ Table 4.15). It is useful when the patient has a limited ability to open the mouth, or when the patient has a strong gag reflex that is elicited by conventional inferior alveolar nerve block.

Injection Technique

- Instruct the patient to close his or her mouth.
- Insert the needle into the mucosa between the medial border of the mandibular ramus and the maxillary tuberosity at the level of the cervical margin of the maxillary molars.
- Advance the needle parallel to the maxillary occlusal plane ~ 20 to 25 mm. At this depth, the tip of the needle should be in the middle of the pterygomandibular space near the inferior alveolar and lingual nerves (▶ Fig. 4.15a, b).
- Following a negative aspiration result, slowly inject the full cartridge of local anesthetic (1.7 mL).

Table 4.15 Anesthesia following an Akinosi block

Areas anesthetized[a] (▶ Fig. 4.15d)	Nerve (▶ Fig. 4.15b)
All mandibular teeth	Inferior alveolar nerve
All buccal gingiva, mucosa, and supporting bone from the second premolar to the central incisor	Mental nerve
All lingual gingiva, mucosa, and supporting bone	Lingual nerve
Anterior two-thirds of the tongue	Lingual nerve
Lower lip	Mental nerve

[a]On the same side as the injection.

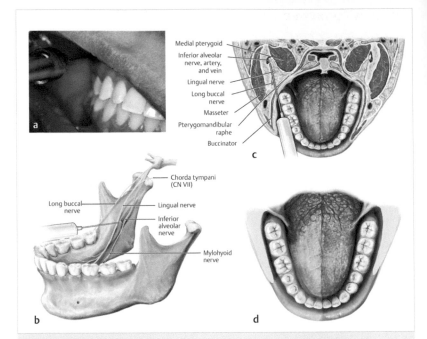

Fig. 4.15 Akinosi block. (**a**) Injection technique. (**b**) Nerves anesthetized, left lateral view. (**c**) Transverse section just above the occlusal plane of the mandibular teeth, superior view. (**d**) Areas anesthetized, superior view. (From Baker EW. Anatomy for Dental Medicine. Illustrations by Voll M and Wesker K. Second Edition. New York: Thieme Medical Publishers; 2015).

Clinical Considerations

- This injection is sufficient for cavity preparations, pulpal procedures, and surgical procedures involving the lingual aspect of the mandibular teeth.
- Extractions of the mandibular molars require supplemental anesthesia of the long buccal nerve.

Long Buccal Nerve Block

Anatomy

The long buccal nerve is a branch of the inferior alveolar nerve (► Table 4.16). It passes along the medial side of the mandibular ramus anterior to the inferior alveolar nerve. It then crosses the anterior border of the mandibular ramus. Its branches innervate the buccal gingiva between the mandibular second premolar and molars, as well as the retromolar triangle

Injection Technique

- Insert the needle into the buccal mucosa posterior to the last molar. It will only penetrate ~ 2 mm (▶ Fig. 4.16**a, b**).
- Following a negative aspiration result, inject ~ 0.5 mL of local anesthetic.

Clinical Considerations

- This injection is used to supplement an inferior alveolar nerve block for extractions or surgical procedures involving the mandibular second premolars to molars.

Table 4.16 Anesthesia following a long buccal nerve block

Areas anesthetized[a] (▶ Fig. 4.16a)	Nerve (▶ Fig. 4.16b)
Buccal gingiva, mucosa, and supporting bone from the mandibular second premolar to the last molar and retromolar trigone	Long buccal nerve (from CN V$_3$)

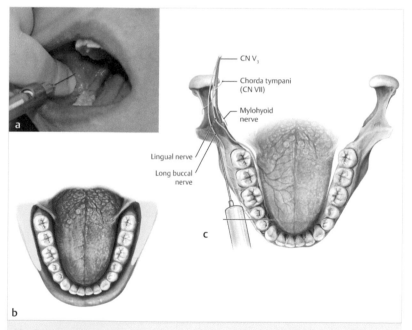

Fig. 4.16 Long buccal nerve block. (**a**) Injection technique. (**b**) Nerves anesthetized, superior view. (**c**) Areas anesthetized, superior view. (From Baker EW. Anatomy for Dental Medicine. Illustrations by Voll M and Wesker K. Second Edition. New York: Thieme Medical Publishers; 2015).

Supplementary Sublingual Nerve Infiltration

Anatomy

The lingual nerve passes downward together with the inferior alveolar nerve and communicates with the chorda tympani of the facial nerve just before reaching the mandibular foramen. This connection gives off secretory fibers to the submandibular and sublingual glands via the submandibular ganglion and taste fibers to the anterior two-thirds of the tongue. The trunk of the lingual nerve gives off branches that innervate the lingual gingiva in the molar region. The lingual gingiva and mucosa of the floor of the mouth are innervated by the sublingual nerve, a branch of the lingual nerve (▸ Table 4.17).

Injection Technique

- Introduce the needle just below the attached gingiva on the lingual side of the tooth requiring lingual anesthesia.
- Following a negative aspiration result, slowly inject a small amount of local anesthetic.

Clinical Considerations

- This injection is used to supplement a mucobuccal fold infiltration or mental nerve block for extractions of the mandibular incisors, canine, and premolar teeth. It is not necessary for extraction of the mandibular molar teeth because the lingual nerve trunk is anesthetized as part of the inferior alveolar block given in these cases.
- Hematoma formation may occur if the injection lacerates the vessels in the floor of the mouth.

Table 4.17 Supplementary sublingual nerve infiltration

Areas anesthetized[a]	Nerve
Lingual gingiva and supporting bone, and the mucosa of the floor of the mouth in the vicinity of the infiltration	Sublingual nerve

[a]On the same side as the injection.

5 Common Oral Lesions

Elizabeth A. Andrews

Introduction

In this chapter, common oral conditions encountered regularly in practice are presented by their name and definition along with applicable alternative names, clinical features, demographics, diagnoses, microscopic features, treatments, and prognoses. Suggested differential diagnoses are provided but are not intended as an exclusive list of all oral entities that should be considered. Each patient case should be assessed for a differential diagnosis that is most fitting for his or her unique presentation.

Developing a Differential Diagnosis

When a lesion is identified upon a thorough head and neck exam, the process taken after identification is also important. The diagnosis and appropriate treatment of abnormal findings may be obvious after the thorough history and examination. Generally, there are various possible diagnoses, therefore a clinical differential diagnosis and plan of investigation needs to be developed.

Possible diagnoses should be recorded in the order of probability based on their prevalence and likelihood of causing the symptoms and signs. Even if only one diagnosis seems like the most appropriate, it is worth noting the next most likely possibility and any other causes that cannot be excluded. Formulating a differential diagnosis helps even experienced clinicians organize their thoughts. Precise diagnosis depends on histological findings.

Appropriate Medical Terminology

Appropriate medical terminology should always be used to describe clinical findings in the records because lay terminology can be misleading and nonspecific. High-quality digital photographs may also be printed and enclosed with the biopsy specimen or can be e-mailed separately to the pathologist. Photographs are helpful in demonstrating the clinical characteristics of the lesion. Box 5.1 lists several common physical descriptions that are useful in describing oral and maxillofacial pathologic entities.

Box 5.1 Descriptive Pathology Terminology

- *Bulla (pl. bullae):* a blister; an elevated, circumscribed, fluid-containing lesion of skin or mucosa.
- *Crusts (crusted):* dried or clotted serum on the surface of the skin or mucosa.
- *Dysplasia (dysplastic):* any abnormal development of cellular size, shape, or organization in tissue.
- *Erosion:* a shallow, superficial ulceration.
- *Hyperkeratosis:* an overgrowth of the cornified layer of epithelium.
- *Hyperplasia (hyperplastic):* an increased number of normal cells.
- *Hypertrophy (hypertrophic):* an increase in size that is caused by an increase in the size of cells not in the number of cells.
- *Keratosis (keratotic):* An overgrowth and thickening of cornified (horned layer) epithelium.
- *Leukoplakia:* a slowly developing change in mucosa characterized by firmly attached, thickened, white patches.
- *Macule:* a circumscribed, nonelevated area of color change that is distinct from adjacent tissues.
- *Malignant:* anaplastic; a cancer that is potentially invasive and metastatic.
- *Nodule:* a large, elevated, circumscribed, solid, palpable mass of the skin or mucosa.
- *Papule:* a small, elevated, circumscribed, solid, palpable mass of the skin or mucosa.
- *Plaque:* a flat, slightly elevated, superficial lesion.
- *Pustule:* a small, cloudy, elevated, circumscribed, pus-containing vesicle on the skin or mucosa.
- *Scale:* a thin, compressed, superficial flake of cornified (keratinized) epithelium.
- *Stomatitis:* any generalized inflammatory condition of the oral mucosa.
- *Ulcer:* a crater-like, circumscribed surface lesion resulting from necrosis of the epithelium.
- *Vesicle:* a small blister; a small, circumscribed elevation of skin or mucosa containing serous fluid.

Leukoplakia

Definition: White (*leuko*) patch (*plakia*)

Alternate names: White plaque, callus, frictional keratosis, dysplasia.

Clinical features: Leukoplakia (▶ Fig. 5.1) is not a histologic diagnosis. It is a clinical description defined by the World Health Organization (WHO) as a "white patch or plaque that cannot be wiped off nor characterized clinically or pathologically as any other disease."

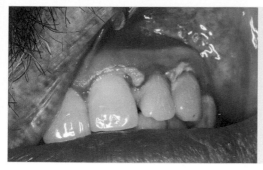

Fig. 5.1 Multiple white leukoplakic plaques on the facial marginal gingiva of the left anterior maxillary teeth.

The oral mucosa can produce a tough protective protein called keratin which, when produced in excess, may appear as a white patch. This mucosal thickening is often part of the tissues' normal protective response against rubbing, pressure, and other forms of local irritation. Other causes may include tobacco use, alcohol abuse, and sun exposure. Histologic diagnoses of biopsied leukoplakias range from hyperkeratosis to dysplasia and, at its worse, carcinoma. Overall, 5 to 25% of leukoplakias are dysplasia or carcinoma, but this likelihood also depends on the location of the lesion. Studies show an overall malignant transformation rate of 4 to 47%.

Demographics: Leukoplakias are the most common oral lesions, representing 23.7% of all oral lesions. Approximately 70% of cases occur in males and are usually seen in older adults over 40 years of age. Approximately 70% of oral leukoplakias are found on the lip vermilion, buccal mucosa, and gingiva. The tongue, lip vermillion, and floor of mouth are considered high-risk sites which account for more than 90% of leukoplakias that prove to be dysplastic or malignant.

Diagnosis: If trauma is the suspected cause of a white (leukoplakia) lesion, the clinician should remove the traumatic etiology and recheck the area in 2 weeks for resolution. If the white lesion is not resolved, then a biopsy is required to establish a definitive diagnosis. Sampling both white lesion and normal mucosa is most helpful in establishing a definitive diagnosis.

Microscopic features: Hyperparakeratotic stratified squamous surface epithelium showing a range of patterns from a regular pattern of maturation with scattered typical mitotic figures in the basal layer (*hyperkeratosis*) to invasive cords and islands of malignant epithelium within the lamina propria (*squamous cell carcinoma*). The underlying connective tissue is usually densely collagenized and can contain scattered chronic inflammatory cells.

Treatment: Remove the etiology (if trauma is suspected) and schedule frequent, regular clinical follow-up appointments. A biopsy of the white lesion may be required to confirm the diagnosis and rule out dysplasia and/or malignancy. In general, any dysplasia located in high-risk locations should be completely removed with long-term follow-up and rebiopsy in the event of recurrence. Squamous cell carcinomas (SCCa) are treated more aggressively depending on the stage of the disease.

Prognosis: Malignant transformation rates of oral leukoplakia range from 0.13 to 17.5%, while the rates of 5-year cumulative malignant transformation range from 1.2 to 14.5%. Some reports found a high incidence of malignant transformation in older patients.

Differential diagnosis:
1. Hyperkeratosis (▶ Fig. 5.2).
2. Dysplasia (▶ Fig. 5.3).
3. SCCa (▶ Fig. 5.4).

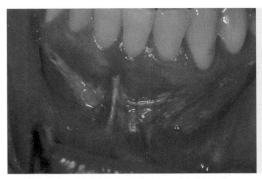

Fig. 5.2 Hyperkeratosis of the anterior mandibular vestibular mucosa.

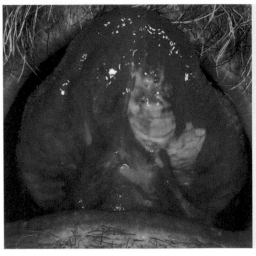

Fig. 5.3 Epithelial dysplasia of the left ventral surface of the tongue.

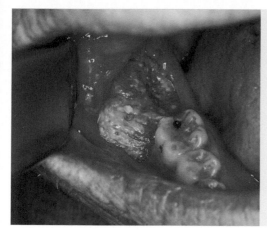

Fig. 5.4 Squamous cell carcinoma of the right posterior mandibular alveolar ridge.

Oral Candidiasis

Definition: An infection of the oral cavity caused by a fungal organism.

Alternate names: Thrush, oral mycosis, moniliasis.

Clinical features: The most common fungal organism present in the oral cavity is *Candida albicans*. This fungal organism is considered a normal component of the oral flora in approximately half of the population. As an opportunist, *Candida* populations will increase in number when the conditions are favorable, resulting in a shift to an infectious presentation. *Candida* infections can appear in various patterns, such as white plaques that scrape off (▶ Fig. 5.5) or red ulcerated areas (▶ Fig. 5.6).

Infections in the oral cavity can range from mild and superficial to severe and disseminated. The clinical presentation is a result of one or more key factors: the host immune status, the environment of the oral cavity, and the type of *C. albicans* present. Patients who wear complete dentures for extended periods of time (e.g., all day and night everyday) have an increased risk of developing candidal infections because the intaglio surface of the dentures provide mucosal coverage and promote a warm, moist environment that is suitable for candidal proliferation. Patients with systemic disorders, such as vitamin B deficiency or anemia, can also present with candidiasis often on the dorsum of the tongue (▶ Fig. 5.7) as a sequela to their underlying disorder.

Diagnosis: Diagnostic exam findings will help a clinician determine the probability of a fungal infection. A clinical finding of a white area that is easily scraped off—resulting in an underlying erythematous base—is highly probable for *Candida* infection. The most specific method for confirming the diagnosis of

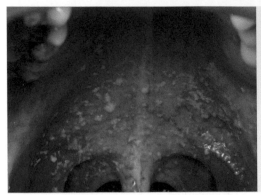

Fig. 5.5 Widespread white candidal plaques across the palatal mucosa.

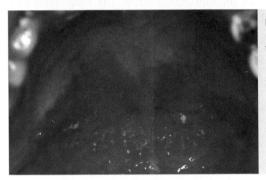

Fig. 5.6 Large erythematous ulcerated candidal infection of the palatal mucosa.

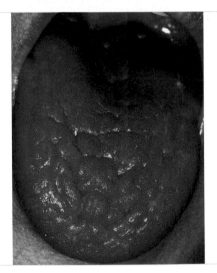

Fig. 5.7 Candidiasis of the dorsum of the tongue in a patient with vitamin B deficiency.

fungal infection is a cytologic smear or a biopsy of the affected tissue submitted for microscopic diagnosis.

Microscopic features: Microscopic analysis of either an exfoliative cytology sample or a biopsy tissue section will reveal candidal hyphae and yeast buds when stained appropriately. When stained with periodic acid–Schiff (PAS) or the Grocott-Gomori methenamine silver (GMS) stains, the candidal hyphae and yeasts are more easily identified. These stains highlight the fungal wall allowing for observable confirmation. The specimen will show numerous fungal organisms consistent with *C. albicans.*

Treatment: The first choice of treatment for oral candidiasis is a polyene agent, such as nystatin or clotrimazole troches. If the patient wears a denture, the denture should also be disinfected and treated in order to ensure complete treatment of the mucosa. This can be accomplished by cleaning the intaglio surface of the denture in 0.12% chlorhexidine solution. The most important aspect of treatment in edentulous patients is to improve denture hygiene. Instruct patients to remove the denture at night and clean/disinfect the prosthesis. The second line of treatment of a persistent infection is a triazole systemic agent such as fluconazole.

Prognosis: Oral candidiasis is typically a condition with no long-term consequences. It usually resolves with patient compliance resulting in improved denture hygiene and/or with proper use of the antifungal medication. In severely immunocompromised patients, the infection may present a more serious threat and persist intermittently for longer periods of time. If confirmed infection does not resolve, a patient should be referred to their primary care provider for a systemic medical work-up and management.

Differential diagnosis:

1. Allergic contact stomatitis (▶ Fig. 5.8).
2. Atrophic lichen planus (▶ Fig. 5.9).
3. Morsicatio buccarum (▶ Fig. 5.10).

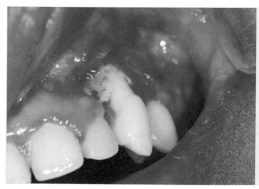

Fig. 5.8 Allergic contact stomatitis of the facial gingiva of the left maxillary canine area. This patient repeatedly placed cinnamon-flavored chewing gum in the buccal vestibule in this area.

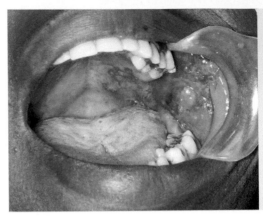

Fig. 5.9 Atrophic lichen planus of the left posterior palate and the left buccal mucosa.

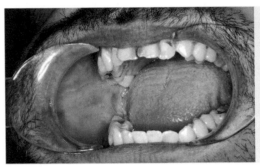

Fig. 5.10 Morsicatio buccarum (chronic cheek biting) of the right buccal mucosa.

Irritation Fibroma

Definition: Exuberant scar tissue.

   Alternate names: Focal fibrous hyperplasia, keloid.

   Clinical features: Irritation fibroma occurs due to acute or repeated trauma to an oral site. The injured area will exhibit poor healing and possibly inflammation in the area of trauma. This may then result in a growth of tissue in response to the repeated trauma. Clinically, the fibroma will be a smooth surfaced, tissue-colored, dome-shaped nodule with a sessile (broad-based) attachment. These are most common on the buccal mucosa and the tongue. Patients often exhibit a parafunctional habit and have no symptoms related to the growth itself. In others, reactive lesions like pyogenic granuloma may fibrose over time into a fibroma. These lesions could demonstrate pigmenta-

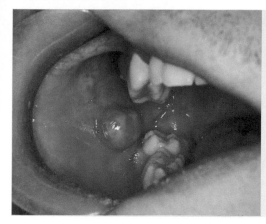

Fig. 5.11 Large (1.5 cm) smooth-surfaced, tissue-colored, dome-shaped fibroma with a sessile (broad) base on the right buccal mucosa.

tions from reactive melanosis or ulcerations if recently traumatized. They usually are smaller than 1 cm in diameter, but may grow to 3 to 4 cm in some patients (▶ Fig. 5.11). These lesions grow slowly, achieve full size within 6 months, and do not resolve on their own.

Demographics: While there is no gender predilection, fibromas typically occur in patients 40 to 60 years old; with a smaller, bimodal distribution in children as well. The lesions occur most commonly on the buccal mucosa, followed by the lip, lateral tongue, and the gingiva. Fibroma is the third most common lesion in adult patients.

Diagnosis: Clinical correlation will indicate that a lesion with this appearance and behavior is most often a fibroma. However, an excisional biopsy is indicated to remove the obvious lesion and confirm the diagnosis histologically.

Microscopic features: Sections will show an exophytic nodule surfaced by hyperparakeratotic, mildly atrophic, stratified squamous epithelium. The relatively avascular underlying connective tissue will contain bundles of dense collagen supporting spindled fibroblasts. Scattered chronic inflammatory cells will also be observed.

Treatment: The definitive treatment is conservative surgical excision and submission of tissue for histopathologic diagnosis.

Prognosis: The prognosis is excellent with excision and elimination of the traumatic etiology.

Differential diagnosis:
1. Neurofibroma (▶ Fig. 5.12).
2. Benign salivary gland neoplasm (▶ Fig. 5.13).
3. Malignant salivary gland neoplasm (▶ Fig. 5.14).

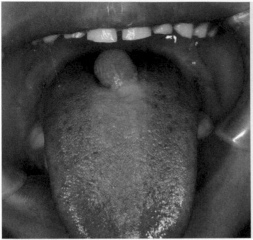

Fig. 5.12 Tissue-colored neurofibroma of the midline dorsum of the tongue.

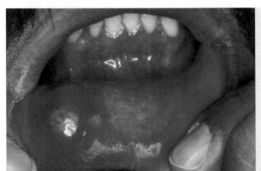

Fig. 5.13 Large (1.7 cm) benign salivary gland neoplasm of the right lower lip mucosa.

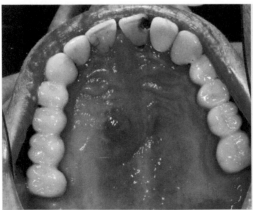

Fig. 5.14 Malignant salivary gland neoplasm of the right palate. The lesion is raised, ulcerated, and firm to palpation.

Squamous Papilloma

Definition: A benign epithelial proliferation that has papillary architecture.

   Alternate names: Papilloma, oral wart.

   Clinical features: These lesions are soft, painless epithelial protrusions that are most often pedunculated and exophytic (▶ Fig. 5.15).

   Papillomas are induced by infection with the human papilloma virus (HPV). The HPV types that cause papillomas are typically those that do not incorporate into the host DNA and pose little risk of malignancy (most commonly HPV 6 and 11). The mode of transmission is through sexual contact—person to person—whereby the virus is inserted into traumatized, exposed epithelium. Clinically, the papilloma has numerous fingerlike surface projections that impart a "cauliflower" or wart-like appearance (▶ Fig. 5.16).

   There is often a latency period of 3 to 12 months before the clinical presentation is observed.

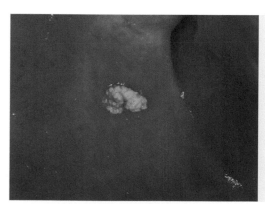

Fig. 5.15 Small (1.0 cm), soft, exophytic, white squamous papilloma of the left soft palate.

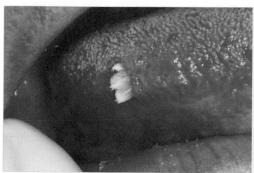

Fig. 5.16 Small papilloma with numerous fingerlike surface projections that impart a "cauliflower" or wart-like appearance on the right lateral tongue.

Demographics: There is no gender predilection, with the typical age range consisting of 30 to 50 years. The most common locations are the tongue, lips, and soft palate. Approximately 1 out of 250 adults are infected with HPV and the papilloma accounts for 3% of all oral biopsies. This lesion, when in the genital region, can be transmitted from mother to child. This type of transmission accounts for approximately 7 to 8% of oral lesions in children.

Diagnosis: In order to diagnose this entity, a surgical excision with submission for microscopic diagnosis is required. DNA analysis can be obtained to ascertain the type of HPV infection present in the tissue.

Microscopic features: A pedunculated mass surfaced by parakeratotic, hyperplastic stratified squamous epithelium arranged in a frond-like configuration showing scattered typical mitotic figures in the parabasal layer. Koilocytes will be present in the spinous layer. The finger-like projections are supported by a thin, vascular, fibrous connective tissue core that also contains scattered chronic inflammatory cells.

Treatment: Surgical excision of the lesion to its base with close clinical follow-up is required. Confirmation of diagnosis predicates frequent surveillance for other papillomas or papillary growths orally and genitally. Preventative measures are in place to decrease the papilloma incidence with the development of vaccinations that target the most common low-risk HPV strains and two high-risk HPV strains.

Prognosis: The prognosis is good with complete removal and counseling regarding etiology in order to prevent further infections. Frequent oral evaluation is important, as high-risk HPV is also an etiologic factor in some oral cancers. Knowledge of previous infections is important to ascertain risk for a high-risk infection.

Differential diagnosis:
1. Verruca vulgaris (▶ Fig. 5.17).
2. Verrucous carcinoma (▶ Fig. 5.18).
3. Condyloma acuminatum (▶ Fig. 5.19).

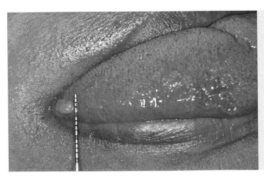

Fig. 5.17 Small, exophytic verruca vulgaris lesion of the right lateral tongue.

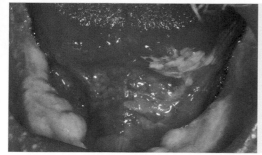

Fig. 5.18 Irregular, raised, and poorly defined verrucous carcinoma white lesion of the left ventral surface of the tongue and floor of mouth.

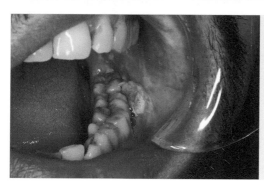

Fig. 5.19 Firm, whitish-pink, exophytic condyloma acuminatum of the left posterior mandibular facial gingiva in the area of the second molar.

Mucocele

Definition: Benign growth that contains a collection of saliva in the parenchymal tissue of the oral cavity.

Alternate names: Mucous retention cyst, mucous extravasation cyst, mucous cyst of the oral mucosa.

Clinical features: Mucoceles are described as soft-tissue swellings that are fluctuant, dome-shaped, smooth-surfaced, and translucent to blue in color (▶ Fig. 5.20).

A common cause is a traumatic severance of a minor salivary gland duct that causes saliva to pool in the connective tissue plane instead of being excreted into the oral cavity. Most patients report a post-traumatic, persistent swelling of an accidentally bitten area. Mucoceles are usually asymptomatic, but at times may be tender. They are described as increasing and decreasing in size throughout the day, especially during meals as salivation is increased.

Demographics: There is no gender predilection and the lesion is usually diagnosed in young patients, including adolescents and teenagers. The most common location is the lower lip.

Diagnosis: In order to diagnose the lesion, a sufficient excisional sample must be procured in order to obtain the entire lesion and, thus, establish a correct diagnosis.

Microscopic features: A nodule surfaced by parakeratotic, stratified squamous epithelium. The lamina propria will exhibit an area of extravasated mucin that is surrounded by a thin granulation tissue wall. Minor salivary glands showing a mild chronic inflammatory cell infiltrate should also be sampled.

Treatment: The best treatment is surgical excision of the affected gland(s). To ensure the best outcome, removal of minor glands around the incision is necessary. There is a low rate of recurrence, but the surgical removal of a mucocele might cut an adjacent duct with a resultant recurrence.

Prognosis: If properly removed, mucoceles have a low recurrence rate and an excellent prognosis.

Differential diagnosis:
1. Salivary gland neoplasm (▶ Fig. 5.21).
2. Fibroma (▶ Fig. 5.22).
3. Hemangioma/varix (▶ Fig. 5.23).

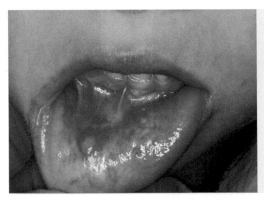

Fig. 5.20 Well-defined, small, raised, dome-shaped, smooth surfaced mucocele of the right lower lip mucosa.

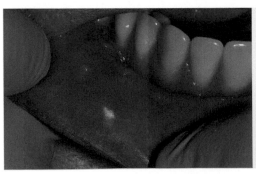

Fig. 5.21 Poorly defined, raised, erythematous salivary gland neoplasm of the right lower lip mucosa.

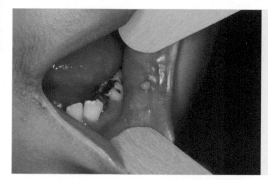

Fig. 5.22 Well-defined, small, firm, tissue-colored, dome-shaped fibroma of the left lower lip/buccal mucosa.

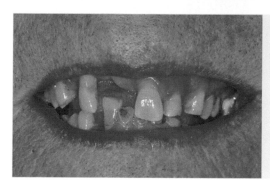

Fig. 5.23 Small, bluish, slightly raised, well-defined heman-gioma/varix slightly left of the midline of the lower lip.

Lichen Planus

Definition: Lichen planus (LP) is a chronic immune-mediated disorder that affects the oral mucosal tissues as well as the dermis. The term *lichen* comes from the clinical appearance that resembles the lichen plants found on rocks.

Alternate names: None

Clinical features: LP is a disorder that affects the oral cavity, the skin, and other mucosal sites in the body. Clinically, the patent will exhibit lesions that may demonstrate a lacy or web-like appearance (reticular type; ► Fig. 5.24) or an irregular white patch.

The white lines will intersect with larger and smaller white lines radiating out from a central clear area. The background mucosa is either normal or slightly erythematous. Typically, the lesions will be bilateral on the buccal mucosa, but may be found on other oral tissues such as the gingiva (► Fig. 5.25) and the tongue.

There are three major subtypes: reticular, the most common form of oral LP, erosive (► Fig. 5.26), and hyperplastic (► Fig. 5.27).

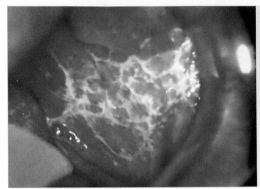

Fig. 5.24 White, striated, lacy, web-like reticular type lichen planus of the left buccal mucosa.

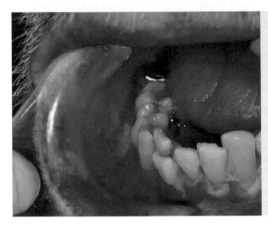

Fig. 5.25 White striations of lichen planus on the anterior and posterior right mandibular facial gingiva.

The lesions will come and go over time without complete resolution. Quite often, the patients will be asymptomatic and unaware of the disorder.

Demographics: Oral LP is common with approximately 3 to 4% of the population exhibiting this disorder. Approximately 25% of patients with dermal LP will have oral lesions, so it is important to examine the dermis when a suspected LP is found in the oral cavity. Over half of the patients with LP are females 40 years of age or older.

Diagnosis: Once lesions are observed, assessment for other lesions on the skin and mucosal sites should be made. Establishing a history of blisters will help determine the next steps for diagnosis. If such a history is present, a biopsy is indicated to rule out other immune-mediated blistering conditions such as pemphigus vulgaris. When performing the biopsy, it is important to

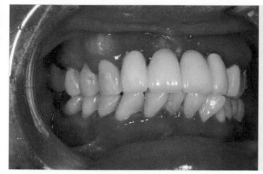

Fig. 5.26 Erosive lichen planus of the right anterior maxillary lateral incisor area and right anterior mandibular facial gingiva.

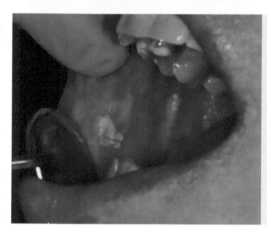

Fig. 5.27 Multiple irregularly shaped, white, flat, and slightly raised hyperplastic lichen planus lesions of the right buccal mucosa.

obtain an area of normal and lesional tissue in the sample. Because this is an immune-mediated disorder, direct immunofluorescence may be necessary to rule out other immune-mediated disorders. If a unilateral presentation is observed, determining a potential insult, such as a drug or restorative materials, behind induced lichenoid reactions remains a key task.

Microscopic features: The specimen will be surfaced by parakeratotic, focally acanthotic, and stratified squamous epithelium showing a regular pattern of maturation. The underlying submucosa will contain a band-like infiltrate comprising lymphocytes, plasma cells, and occasional mast cells and eosinophils. Destruction of the epithelial–connective tissue junction will be visible, but is actually an artifact of the immune process. The rete pegs will exhibit a saw-toothed appearance. There is often a mild exocytosis of lymphocytes into the epithelium.

Treatment: There is no cure for LP. In the reticular subtype, no treatment is needed. In the erosive subtype, topical corticosteroids may be applied to alleviate the symptoms.

Antifungal therapy should be considered when associated with a burning sensation, as a fungal organism may overgrow in the aftermath of steroid application. All lesions should be assessed regularly—with 6-month evaluations—for changes that are consistent with dysplasia or other precancerous entities.

Prognosis: There is a slight—less than 1%—increase in the risk of developing SCCa in LP patients. The prognosis nonetheless remains good for most patients with proper control of symptoms.

Differential diagnosis:

1. Lichenoid mucositis (▶ Fig. 5.28).
2. Lupus erythematosus (▶ Fig. 5.29).
3. Pemphigus (▶ Fig. 5.30).

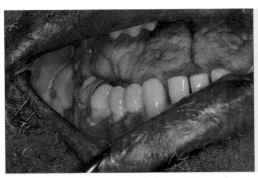

Fig. 5.28 Ill-defined erythematous lichenoid mucositis of the right mandibular facial gingiva in the premolar-molar region.

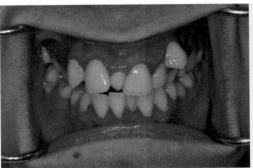

Fig. 5.29 Lupus erythematosus affecting the maxillary and mandibular marginal gingiva. Note the linear band of gingival erythema.

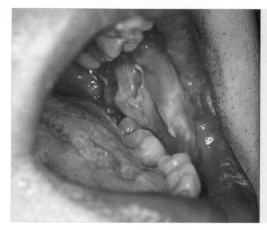

Fig. 5.30 Several painful pemphigus vulgaris ulcerations covered with fibrin of the left buccal mucosa.

Pyogenic Granuloma

Definition: The name, if taken literally, does not accurately describe this lesion. It is not an infection, does not produce pus as the term "pyogenic" suggests, and is not a granulomatous infection. This lesion is formed during the normal healing process due to a deficiency in the reduction of granulation tissue after irritation or trauma.

Alternate names: Eruptive hemangioma, granulation tissue-type hemangioma, lobular capillary hemangioma, pregnancy tumor.

Clinical features: The pyogenic granuloma (PG) presents as a painless erythematous mass that is often hemorrhagic when palpated (▶ Fig. 5.31).

Quite often, it will be lobulated and/or ulcerated at its surface. The attachment is either sessile or pedunculated. Typically, the lesion is painless and is only discovered because it bleeds upon brushing. Some PG will grow rapidly causing concern for a possible malignancy (▶ Fig. 5.32).

In addition to a traditional PG, two specialized variants may occur under specific circumstances. The pregnancy tumor, also known as epulis gravidarum, is a PG subtype in pregnant women that often self-resolves upon childbirth. Epulis granulomatosum is a PG growth within an extraction socket (▶ Fig. 5.33 and ▶ Fig. 5.34).

Demographics: This lesion is more commonly seen in children and young adults. It occurs on the gingiva in 75% of cases, but can otherwise be found on the lips, tongue, and buccal mucosa. This is the 50th most common oral mucosal lesion diagnosed in patients and is present in approximately 1:10,000 adults.

Diagnosis: Clinical correlation along with complete excision of the tissue with submission for microscopic evaluation will confirm the diagnosis of a PG.

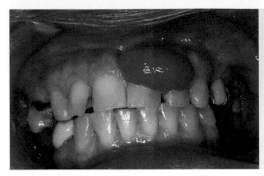

Fig. 5.31 Painless, erythematous pyogenic granuloma on the maxillary left anterior gingiva.

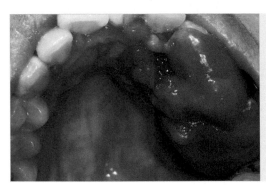

Fig. 5.32 Large, erythematous, rapidly growing pyogenic granuloma covering most of the maxillary left dentition.

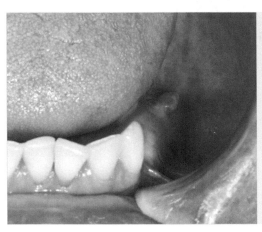

Fig. 5.33 Exophytic erythematous epulis granulomatosum within and emerging from an extraction socket in the left mandibular molar area.

Microscopic features: The lesion is surfaced by parakeratotic stratified squamous epithelium showing a loss of continuity that is replaced by a fibrinopurulent membrane. The lamina propria is composed of highly vascular connective tissue in a semilobular arrangement with numerous endothelial-lined channels filled with erythrocytes. A mixed inflammatory cell infiltrate comprising neutrophils, lymphocytes, histiocytes, and plasma cells is present.

Treatment: Its treatment is surgical excision to the base and removal of the cause of the growth. In the instance of a pregnancy tumor, it is usually best to wait until after the birth of the child, as the PG may shrink or disappear once the child is born.

Prognosis: The prognosis is good, but PGs may recur if the original cause is not removed or if more infection or trauma is introduced to the area.

Differential diagnosis:
1. Peripheral ossifying fibroma (▶ Fig. 5.35).
2. Peripheral giant cell granuloma (▶ Fig. 5.36).
3. Metastatic tumor (▶ Fig. 5.37 and ▶ Fig. 5.38).

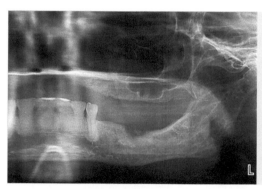

Fig. 5.34 Shallow left mandibular molar extraction socket and crestal alveolar bony concavity deep to the epulis granulomatosum shown in ▶ Fig. 5.33.

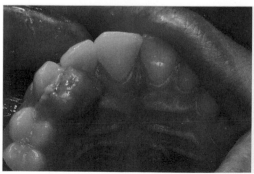

Fig. 5.35 Firm, pink, broad-based peripheral ossifying fibroma on the right maxillary palatal gingiva adjacent to the canine.

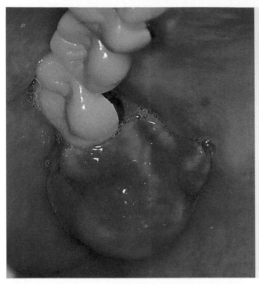

Fig. 5.36 Firm, pink, pedunculated peripheral giant cell granuloma on the right maxillary palatal gingiva.

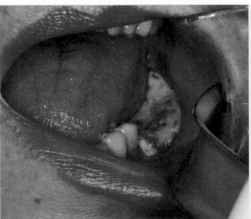

Fig. 5.37 Large ulcerated metastatic breast cancer mass of the left posterior mandibular body.

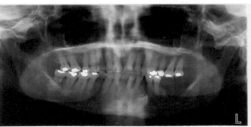

Fig. 5.38 Poorly defined, diffuse, osteolytic metastatic breast cancer lesion of the left mandibular body. This is the radiographic appearance of the lesion seen in ▶ Fig. 5.37.

Oral Ulceration

Definition: An ulceration is an area devoid of overlying epithelium. Ulcerations can be caused by many different factors. For example, a traumatic ulceration develops secondary to a trauma, such as cheek biting or tongue biting.

Alternate names: Traumatic ulcer, traumatic ulcerative granuloma with stromal eosinophilia (TUGSE), nonspecific ulcer, herpetic ulceration.

Clinical features: Ulcerations may manifest clinically in several ways. Most often, they appear as a well-defined, slightly depressed lesion. The center is often erythematous to yellow and may have an irregular white halo which can manifest as rolled borders. Sometimes ulcerations appear to have a yellowish center that represents a thick fibrinopurulent membrane (▶ Fig. 5.39). This fibrin membrane can be removed with a firm sweeping motion.

It is not always possible to differentiate between traumatic ulcerations and other ulcerations, such as oral aphthae (▶ Fig. 5.40) based on clinical or microscopic appearance.

A subtype of traumatic ulceration termed traumatic ulcerative granuloma with stromal eosinophilia (TUGSE) also exists in which a large number of eosinophils are present (▶ Fig. 5.41).

TUGSE may be raised and ulcerated with rolled margins mimicking the presentation of SCCa. While the presumed cause behind TUGSE is trauma, a corresponding history may not always be present indicating a multifactorial etiology. Ulcerations that are of viral etiology, specifically herpetic lesions (▶ Fig. 5.42), should also be considered and excluded based on history and the location of the ulceration.

Other infectious agents, such as fungal entities, also remain possible causes. Clinical correlation is necessary and should be provided to the pathologist when a biopsy sample is submitted.

Demographics: There is no gender predilection with ulcerations. Location, age, and prevalence will be specific to the etiology of the ulcer.

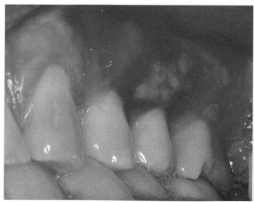

Fig. 5.39 Moderately sized, well-demarcated traumatic ulceration on the left maxillary facial gingiva.

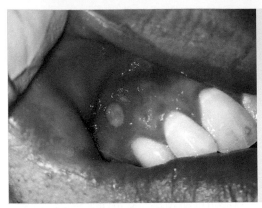

Fig. 5.40 Small, erythematous, noncontagious, ovoid aphthous ulceration with well-circumscribed borders on the right maxillary facial gingiva.

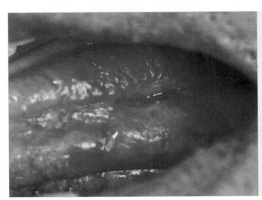

Fig. 5.41 Left lateral surface of the tongue traumatic ulcerative granuloma with stromal eosinophilia (TUGSE).

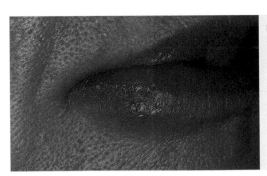

Fig. 5.42 Right lower lip herpes labialis lesion (cold sore).

Diagnosis: Definitive diagnosis of an ulceration can only be made with a scalpel or tissue punch biopsy. An adequate biopsy will include both a portion of the ulceration and adjacent nonulcerated tissue. The differential diagnosis of an ulceration includes serious conditions such as SCCa. Therefore, the standard of care is to biopsy an ulceration if it has not resolved in 2 weeks. It is in the patient's best interest to submit oral tissues to oral and maxillofacial pathologists who, in contrast to general pathologists, have acquired extensive training in the diagnosis of oral lesions. This will ensure the most accurate diagnosis is rendered.

Microscopic features: By definition, an ulceration lacks overlying epithelium. A mix of acute inflammation and fibrin, termed a fibrinopurulent membrane, usually covers the underlying connective tissue. Beneath this membrane is the ulcer bed which is composed of inflamed granulation tissue. The adjacent epithelium may be covered by increased keratin or parakeratin in an attempt to protect the epithelium. The epithelium may even exhibit atypia secondary to the reactive process. Sometimes it is difficult or impossible to distinguish if the atypia present is reactive or is secondary to a premalignant process termed epithelial dysplasia.

Treatment: After clinical identification of an ulceration, the first step is to identify and eliminate the source(s) of trauma, if a mechanical insult is suspected. In the setting of an edentulous patient, the source of trauma may be an ill-fitting denture. Other sources of irritation may include hard foods (crusty bread, chips with sharper edges, etc.) or parafunctional habits such as cheek- or tongue-biting. Infectious etiologies such as herpes viruses, immune-mediated causes such as aphthae, and habit-based causes such as tobacco use are also important considerations.

Prognosis: With identification and removal of the local irritating factor(s), the lesion should resolve in 2 weeks without consequence. If an ulceration has not resolved in 2 weeks, the standard of care is to biopsy the lesion to establish a definitive diagnosis and rule out the possibility of a developing SCCa or other malignancies.

Differential diagnosis:
1. TUGSE (▶ Fig. 5.43).
2. Herpes virus (▶ Fig. 5.44).
3. Aphthous stomatitis (▶ Fig. 5.45).
4. SCCa (▶ Fig. 5.46)

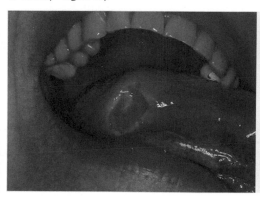

Fig. 5.43 Right lateral tongue traumatic ulcerative granuloma with stromal eosinophilia (TUGSE).

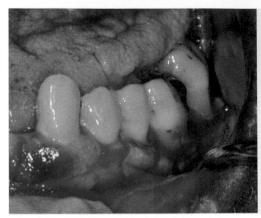

Fig. 5.44 Symptomatic herpetic gingivostomatitis ulcerations of the left mandibular molar facial gingiva.

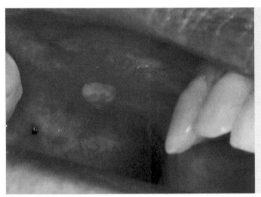

Fig. 5.45 Symptomatic minor aphthous ulceration (canker sore) of the right posterior maxillary vestibular mucosa.

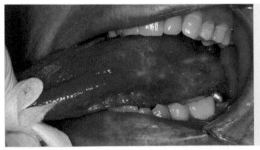

Fig. 5.46 Left ventrolateral tongue poorly defined, diffuse, indurated mixed red-white squamous cell carcinoma lesion.

Amalgam Tattoo

Definition: An iatrogenic discoloration of the mucosa from localized implantation of amalgam material in the tissue.

Alternate names: Focal argyrosis, localized argyrosis.

Clinical features: Amalgam tattoo appears as a pigmented macule that is gray, brown, or black in color (▶ Fig. 5.47).

Clinically, these lesions will be flat or slightly raised with diffuse, ill-defined or well-defined borders. The most common locations for amalgam tattoos are the gingiva, alveolar/buccal mucosa, and the tongue. Bright amalgam particles are sometimes visible on a radiograph if the particles are large enough. Amalgam and other foreign materials can enter the tissue and stain it after trauma to the oral mucosal tissues. This can occur in either the soft tissue or bone. Tattooing may occur as a result of fine particles or dust from mechanical abrasion (often from floss or a bur), which causes visible discoloration of the mucosa. Larger pieces of restorative materials may also enter the bone during extractions or surgical endodontics. Other diagnoses such as oral focal melanosis, medication-induced oral pigmentation, and most importantly, melanoma, must be ruled out.

Demographics: This lesion is common and is found in up to 1% of all patients. When compared to other pigmented etiologies, it is the most common localized pigmentation in the oral cavity.

Diagnosis: Its diagnosis may be conducted clinically as long as reasonable evidence of amalgam exists—radiographically, positionally, or otherwise—in the lesion. It is important to assess all pigmented lesions with diascopy to rule out a vascular lesion and obtain a radiograph of the area to positively identify amalgam particles. If the radiograph is not indicative of amalgam, then a biopsy is indicated to rule out melanoma.

Microscopic features: Sections will demonstrate a strip of mucosa surfaced by a parakeratinized stratified squamous epithelium showing a normal pattern of maturation. The lamina propria will exhibit black foreign material consistent

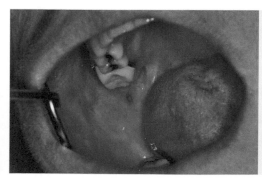

Fig. 5.47 Small (< 1.0 cm), well-defined, flat, bluish-black amalgam tattoo of the right posterior buccal mucosa.

with dental amalgam. This foreign material elicits a mild chronic inflammatory cell response and stains reticulin fibers surrounding vascular channels.

Treatment: If the amalgam is visible within the soft tissue on a radiograph, then no treatment is necessary. However, if it is not visible then a biopsy is indicated to confirm the clinical diagnosis and to rule out melanoma.

Prognosis: Long-term prognosis is excellent as the material is inert and will cause no harm to the patient. Esthetics often will be the reason a patient will elect to remove the lesion.

Differential diagnosis:
1. Oral melanotic macule (▶ Fig. 5.48).
2. Melanocytic nevus (▶ Fig. 5.49).
3. Melanoma (▶ Fig. 5.50).

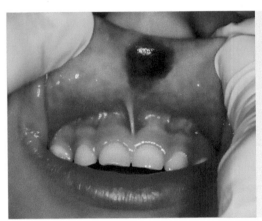

Fig. 5.48 Large (> 1.0 cm), well-defined, slightly raised, pigmented oral melanotic macule on the labial surface of the upper lip in a pediatric patient.

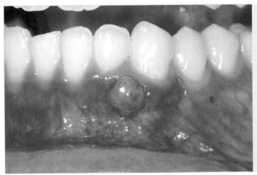

Fig. 5.49 Small, well-defined, slightly raised, pigmented melanocytic nevus on the labial gingiva in the left mandibular canine-lateral incisor area.

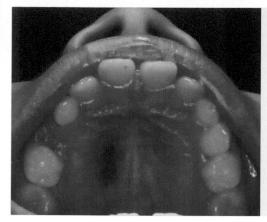

Fig. 5.50 Moderately sized, flat, pigmented melanoma of the right hard palatal mucosa.

Nasopalatine Duct Cyst

Definition: Developmental fissural cyst located adjacent to the incisive canal.

Alternate names: Incisive canal cyst.

Clinical features: This lesion is a developmental cyst that occurs when epithelial remnants of the nasopalatine duct are entrapped in lines of fusion of the palatal bones during development. Clinically, it occurs in the median of the palate—usually anterior to first molars and between the roots of the maxillary central incisors. The lesion may only be noted on a routine radiograph, as it often does not cause symptoms. Its appearance is associated with a teardrop or heart-shaped radiolucency, commonly between the roots of the maxillary central incisors (▶ Fig. 5.51).

In some cases, there may be a smooth swelling of the anterior hard palate, where the swelling may be associated with fluid drainage as well as an expansion of the surrounding tissue. Some patients will report pain in the area, but most often there are no associated symptoms.

Demographics: The nasopalatine duct cyst (NPDC) occurs most commonly in patients 40 to 60 years of age, with a higher frequency in males compared to females. This cyst is the most common nonodontogenic cyst of the oral cavity with 1% of the patients receiving this diagnosis.

Diagnosis: The diagnosis is established by clinical correlation and biopsy confirmation.

Microscopic features: The specimen consists of a cystic structure lined by cuboidal to pseudostratified ciliated columnar epithelium showing a regular pattern of maturation. The cyst wall will be densely collagenized and supports a mild chronic inflammatory cell infiltrate and plump, spindled fibroblasts. Numerous thick- and thin-walled vascular channels and portions of non-decalcified bone are present. Portions of peripheral nerve are also identified.

83

Treatment: After determining vitality of the adjacent teeth, the treatment requires surgical enucleation of the cyst with submission of the tissue for histopathologic examination.

Prognosis: The prognosis for the NPDC is excellent with minimal incidence of recurrence.

Differential diagnosis:
1. Salivary gland neoplasm (▶ Fig. 5.52 and ▶ Fig. 5.53).
2. Odontogenic tumor (▶ Fig. 5.54).
3. Periapical cyst (▶ Fig. 5.55).

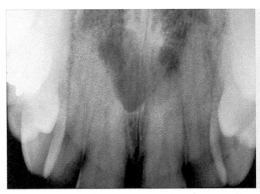

Fig. 5.51 Midline heart-shaped radiolucency between the roots of the maxillary central incisors that is consistent with nasopalatine duct cyst.

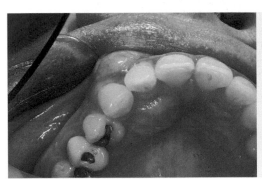

Fig. 5.52 Anterior maxillary facial and palatal swelling caused by a salivary gland neoplasm.

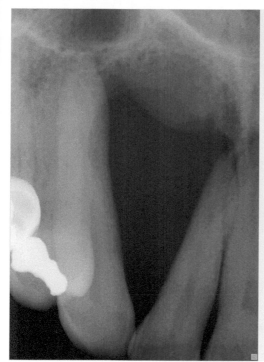

Fig. 5.53 Teardrop radiolucency radiographic appearance of the salivary gland neoplasm shown in ▶ Fig. 5.52.

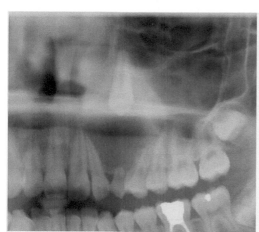

Fig. 5.54 Adenomatoid odontogenic tumor of the left anterior maxilla in the area of the lateral incisor and canine teeth.

85

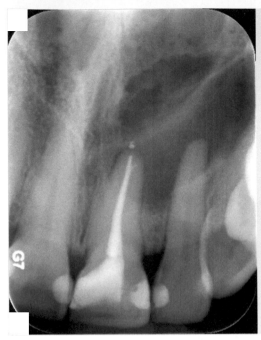

Fig. 5.55 Periapical cyst unilocular radiolucency noted at the apices of the left maxillary central and lateral incisors.

Dentigerous Cyst

Definition: A developmental cyst that forms due to proliferation of the reduced enamel epithelium and a separation of the dental follicle from the developing crown.

Alternate names: Follicular cyst, odontogenic cyst.

Clinical features: The radiographic presentation typically consists of a well-demarcated, unilocular radiolucency surrounding the crown of an impacted tooth (▶ Fig. 5.56).

The unilocular presentation is typically accompanied by a thin sclerotic rim. In large lesions, the teeth may be displaced, roots resorbed, and other dentition impacted. Still, most cases are incidental findings on routine exams with no symptoms reported by the patient.

Demographics: The dentigerous cyst occurs equally in males and females with a typical age between 10 and 30 years. The most common location is around the mandibular third molars followed by the maxillary canines.

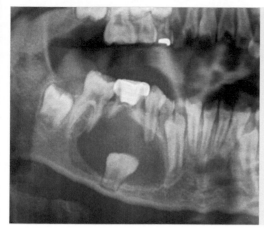

Fig. 5.56 Well-demarcated, unilocular, radiolucent dentigerous cyst surrounding the crown of the impacted mandibular right second premolar.

Dentigerous cyst is the most common developmental cyst and the second most common cyst overall in the oral cavity.

Diagnosis: Enucleation and submission of the tissue for histologic diagnosis in small nonexpansile lesions is required. In large expansile lesions, an *incisional* biopsy is required first to determine the diagnosis in order to plan the optimum treatment, which might include initial decompression/marsupialization. Caution is advised, as more aggressive odontogenic lesions may resemble dentigerous cysts.

Microscopic features: The specimen shows a central cavity partially lined by a thin layer of nonkeratinized stratified squamous epithelium. The connective tissue wall is densely collagenized and contains chronic inflammatory cells that are mainly lymphocytes and plasma cells.

Treatment: Its treatment involves cyst enucleation and, often, extraction of the associated impacted tooth. Marsupialization may be recommended in larger lesions to shrink them prior to removal.

Prognosis: Prognosis is excellent with minimal recurrence. Possible complications are related to potential neoplastic transformation of the cystic epithelium.

Differential diagnosis:
1. Odontogenic keratocyst (▶ Fig. 5.57).
2. Ameloblastoma (▶ Fig. 5.58).
3. Other odontogenic tumors.

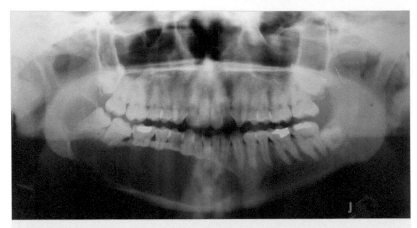

Fig. 5.57 Large, well-demarcated, unilocular odontogenic keratocyst of the right mandible.

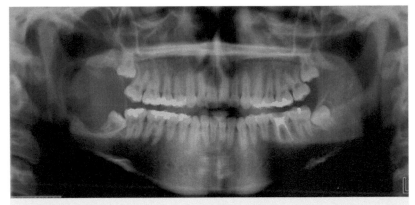

Fig. 5.58 Well-demarcated, unilocular, radiolucent ameloblastoma associated with the crown of the impacted right mandibular third molar.

Bibliography

[1] Regezi JA, Sciubba J, Jordan R. Oral Pathology. 6th ed. W.B. Saunders Company, 2011
[2] Chi A, Neville B, Damm D, Allen C. Oral and Maxillofacial Pathology. 4th ed. Saunders, 2015
[3] Ellis E III. Principles of differential diagnosis and biopsy. In: Hupp JR, Ellis E III, Tucker MR, eds. Contemporary Oral and Maxillofacial Surgery. 6th ed. Mosby, 2014
[4] Kramer IR, Lucas RB, Pindborg JJ, Sobin LH. Definition of leukoplakia and related lesions: an aid to studies on oral precancer. Oral Surg Oral Med Oral Pathol. 1978; 46(4):518–539

[5] Amagasa T, Yamashiro M, Ishikawa H. Oral leukoplakia related to malignant transformation. Oral Sci Int. 2006; 3(2):45–55

[6] Camisasca DR, Silami MA, Honorato J, Dias FL, de Faria PA, Lourenço SdeQ. Oral squamous cell carcinoma: clinicopathological features in patients with and without recurrence. ORL J Otorhinolaryngol Relat Spec. 2011; 73(3):170–176

[7] Genden EM, Ferlito A, Silver CE, et al. Contemporary management of cancer of the oral cavity. Eur Arch Otorhinolaryngol. 2010; 267(7):1001–1017

6 Essentials of Dental Radiographic Analysis and Interpretation

Setareh Lavasani

Introduction

Dentists prescribe multiple radiographic examinations in daily practice to complement clinical examinations and to help reach the most accurate diagnoses. While patients rely on dentists' professional competency and judgment in interpreting those images, extracting the required information is often complicated by the complexity of two-dimensional (2D) representation of three-dimensional (3D) anatomical structures unless the interpreter maintains in-depth familiarity or receives advanced training in oral and maxillofacial radiology.

In addition to 2D images, the recent introduction of 3D cone beam computed tomography (CBCT) enables the dental provider to visualize a more complete picture of structures and pathologies of the head and neck area in all dimensions. While this is a great advantage, it adds a level of complexity of dealing with 3D images and emphasizes the importance of the principles of radiographic interpretation to effectively diagnose pathologies and recognize the incidental findings that are present in the 3D scans.

The purpose of this chapter is to demonstrate the systematic mental steps that an oral and maxillofacial radiologist takes when he/she examines a dental radiograph. Fortunately, radiographic appearances of most oral and maxillofacial pathologies have strong correlations with the lesion's pathophysiology. Vigilance is nonetheless necessary because not all lesions follow typical clinical or radiographic behavior as described in literature.

The steps mentioned in this chapter are intended as suggestions for a thorough, step-by-step systematic approach to reviewing radiographs for logical differential diagnoses. However, providers must remain cognizant of the great variety of possible disease processes and consider consulting an oral and maxillofacial radiologist.

Normal Anatomy

- Knowledge of normal anatomical landmarks, their location/s, and their various presentations is important.
- This reduces the number of "false alarm" diagnoses that can cost the patient time and resources while reducing the dentist's credibility as a competent practitioner.
- Some of the most common normal anatomy variations that are sometimes misdiagnosed as pathology are discussed in subsequent text.

Take a look at the panoramic image below (▶ Fig. 6.1):
- There is a well-defined corticated radiolucency located inferior to the lower border of the left mandibular canal.
- This is a typical location and appearance for the submandibular gland depression, which is a depression caused by the presence of the submandibular gland on the lingual aspect of the mandible.
- Submandibular gland tissue may be found in the depression.

▶ Fig. 6.2 shows a 3D volume rendering from CBCT data.
- In this case, radiographic evaluation and diagnosis help eliminate the need for surgical biopsy and/or further imaging studies.

Other normal anatomical landmarks, such as the incisive foramen, are sometimes present in the area of the midline between the maxillary central incisors and should not be mistaken for an abnormality unless the dimensions are larger than a certain size or if they are causing damage (resorption or displacement) to surrounding structures (such as teeth roots). ▶ Fig. 6.3 demonstrates a normal incisive canal while ▶ Fig. 6.4 demonstrates an incisive canal cyst.
- ▶ Fig. 6.4 shows apical root lateral displacement secondary to the cystic lesion.
- This root displacement is absent in a normal incisive canal.

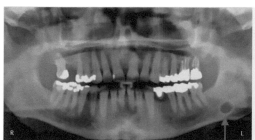

Fig. 6.1 Panoramic radiograph demonstrating a well-defined corticated radiolucency inferior to the lower border of the left mandibular canal (Stafne defect).

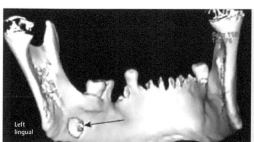

Fig. 6.2 Three-dimensional volume rendering from CBCT data demonstrating a left mandibular lingual cortical bone defect (Stafne defect).

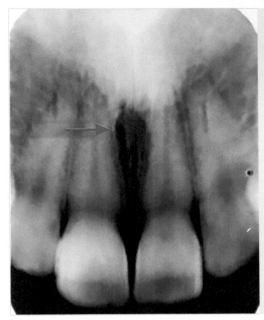

Fig. 6.3 Plain film radiograph demonstrating a normal incisive canal with no apical root displacement of the central incisors.

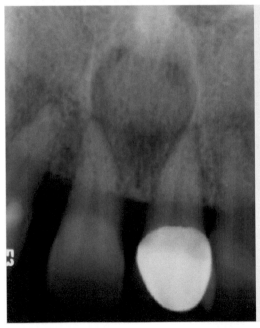

Fig. 6.4 Plain film radiograph demonstrating apical root lateral displacement secondary to an incisive canal cyst.

Symmetry

- When evaluating radiographs, first consider symmetry.
- For example, while evaluating a panoramic radiograph, start from the outer structures, such as the temporomandibular joints (TMJs), and compare both sides.
  - Are both condyles of the same size?
  - Are they of the same shape?
  - Do the joints show signs of osteoarthritic changes, such as flattening of the condylar heads?
  - Does each condyle show the same degree of wear and tear, or does one side show more significant condylar (head) flattening?
  - Does one side look normal while the other side exhibits significant destruction?
- If there is a severe discrepancy in size, shape, or cortication between the two sides, consider what other processes or pathologies may be occurring.

Consider the appearance of the TMJs in the panoramic radiograph shown in
► Fig. 6.5.
- Compare the condylar head, glenoid fossa, and articular eminences' size, shape, and cortication on both sides (bilaterally).
  - Consider that just as all four tires of a car work equally by rotating together simultaneously, similarly the (bilateral) TMJs work simultaneously in equal amounts in opening and closing movements.
  - In doing so, they are expected to have a somewhat similar amount of wear and tear.

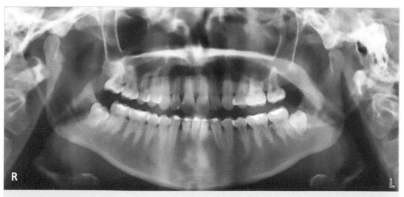

Fig. 6.5 Panoramic radiograph demonstrating relative symmetry of the condylar heads, glenoid fossa, and articular eminences bilaterally.

In the panoramic radiograph below (▶ Fig. 6.6) compare the condylar heads.

- The condyle on the patient's right shows a continuous cortication and minimal bony changes.
- The condylar head on the left side shows destruction of the cortex with a large round radiolucent area.
- This indicates that a different process other than normal wear and tear (other than osteoarthritic changes) should be considered.
- To better evaluate the TMJ in 3D, small volume CBCT scans of the right and left sides should be acquired and evaluated (▶ Fig. 6.7).

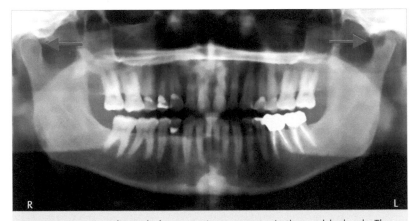

Fig. 6.6 Panoramic radiograph demonstrating asymmetry in the condylar heads. The right condyle shows continuous cortication while the left shows destruction of the cortex.

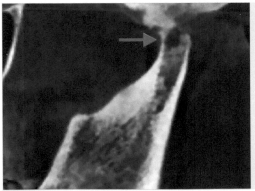

Fig. 6.7 Small volume CBCT scan of the left temporomandibular joint demonstrating destruction of the cortical outline with possible bone-on-bone contact of the condyle with the glenoid fossa and the articular eminence.

- Noting that this example demonstrates unilateral joint damage, the practitioner needs to consider other conditions that could affect the TMJ unilaterally.
  - Systemic medical conditions such as rheumatoid arthritis—an autoimmune disease that could affect different joints in the body unilaterally—ought to be ruled out.
  - Consider a referral to the patient's primary medical doctor for assistance in working up medical conditions that pose risks for unilateral joint changes.
- This case demonstrates that systemic medical conditions may have effects on oral and maxillofacial structures and that dentists may be the first to recognize such conditions.

Mucous Retention (Antral) Pseudocyst

- Evaluate for symmetry when examining the right and left maxillary sinuses.
  - Are the sinuses totally radiolucent or do they display shadows of radiopacity?
  - Evaluate the floors of both maxillary sinuses for integrity and uniformity.
  - If there is a soft tissue shadow (radiopacity) in either maxillary sinus, further examine and try to determine whether the pathology has *grown into* the sinus (elevated floor of the sinus) or if it has *originated from* the maxillary sinus and the floor is being pushed or interrupted.

Consider the panoramic radiograph in ▶ Fig. 6.8.
- The right maxillary sinus exhibits a well-defined dome-shaped soft tissue opacity on the floor of the sinus.

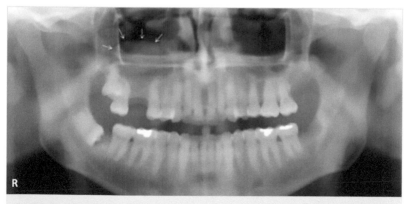

Fig. 6.8 Panoramic radiograph demonstrating a well-defined dome-shaped soft-tissue opacity on the floor of the right maxillary sinus.

- The cortical boundaries and outline of the right maxillary sinus appear to be intact and can be followed for integrity.
  - This demonstrates an example of a mucous retention (antral) pseudocyst, which is a common finding and is the result of a collection and entrapment of mucus in the maxillary sinuses.
  - It is called a pseudocyst because it lacks epithelial lining, and, hence, is not a true cyst.
- With an antral pseudocyst, there is integrity of the medial wall, lateral wall, and floor of the maxillary sinus, which confirms that the lesion is originating *within* the maxillary sinus and does not have aggressive behavior (intact and smooth walls).

Sinus Pathology

- In addition to the benign and self-limiting mucous retention (antral) pseudocyst, the sinuses may contain a variety of other pathologies, such as inflammatory, neoplastic, and/or dysplastic lesions.
- When formulating an accurate differential diagnosis, the first step toward distinguishing the various types of lesions from each other is to follow the cortication of the sinus walls and floor to look for signs that suggest changes in the boundaries.
  - For example, a localized elevation of the floor of the maxillary sinus that is causing opacification of the sinus at the area of an endodontically treated maxillary tooth suggests an odontogenic pathology that is causing inflammation in the sinus mucosa.
  - This may cause mucosal thickening and opacification, as shown in ▶ Fig. 6.9.

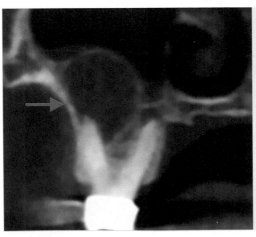

Fig. 6.9 Cone beam computed tomography image demonstrating localized elevation of the floor of the right maxillary sinus caused by the periapical lesion of the right maxillary molar.

Note the localized elevation of the floor of the right maxillary sinus by inflammatory products that are produced in the periapical lesion of the right maxillary molar tooth. Contrast this to the antral pseudocyst where the floor of the maxillary sinus was in place and had not been pushed inward or outward.

Pattern of Radiographic Changes

- In addition to evaluating radiographic images for symmetry in shape and size, it is also important to examine and compare the trabecular and cortical bone patterns in different areas of the image.

In the panoramic reconstructed CBCT image of ▶ Fig. 6.10, evaluate and compare the right and left sides of the jaw in a 38-year-old female patient.
- Note that the pattern of bone trabeculation is different on the right and left sides.
- A normal appearing bone pattern is seen on the left side.
- A ground glass and cotton wool appearing bone pattern is seen on the right side.
- The right mandible appears to be larger than the left side with thickening of the inferior cortex of the right mandible (▶ Fig. 6.11).
- Also note superior displacement of the right mandibular canal to the area near the crest of the right posterior mandibular alveolar ridge and unilateral bodily expansion of the right mandible.
- The demographic, clinical, and CBCT imaging findings of this 38-year-old female combine to present a total "picture" that suggests a type of fibro-osseous lesion such as fibrous dysplasia or Paget's disease of bone.
- Given the unilateral involvement of the bone (*usually seen in fibrous dysplasia*) and the patient's age (*Paget's disease is usually seen in older male patients*), one can reasonably formulate a provisional radiographic diagnosis of fibrous dysplasia.

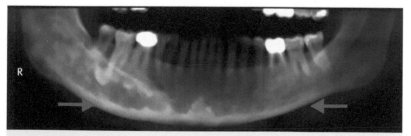

Fig. 6.10 Panoramic reconstructed cone beam computed tomography image of a 38-year-old female demonstrating asymmetry in the bone trabeculation and size of the mandible.

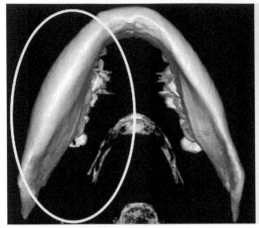

Fig. 6.11 Three-dimensional volume rendering (worm's eye view) demonstrating unilateral bodily expansion and enlargement of the right mandible.

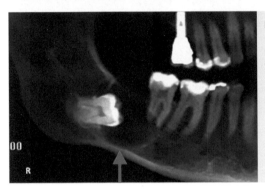

Fig. 6.12 Panoramic reconstructed cone beam computed tomography image demonstrating a pericoronal radiolucent lesion that has displaced the mandibular canal inferiorly.

Location

- When evaluating whether a lesion is of odontogenic, neural, or vascular origin, it is important to pay close attention to its location.
- In general, lesions that form superior to the mandibular canal demonstrate a higher probability of possessing an odontogenic origin.
- This is because the remnants of odontogenic cells that can give rise to odontogenic cysts and tumors are more likely to be found superior to the mandibular canal.

The examples below require close attention to the boundaries of the lesions and their associations with the impacted third molars.

▶ Fig. 6.12 demonstrates a pericoronal radiolucent lesion of odontogenic origin (dentigerous cyst) that has displaced the mandibular canal inferiorly.

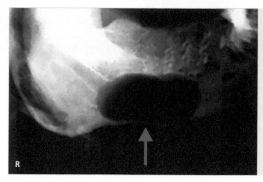

Fig. 6.13 Panoramic radiograph demonstrating a unilocular radiolucency residing within the mandibular canal. This is a neurofibroma.

▶ Fig. 6.13 demonstrates a unilocular radiolucency that appears to reside within the boundaries of the mandibular canal. Considering that the main components of the mandibular canal are neural (inferior alveolar nerve) and vascular (inferior alveolar artery), the lesion within the mandibular canal has a very high probability of being of neural or vascular origin. The example shown in ▶ Fig. 6.13 is a neurofibroma, a benign tumor of neural origin.

Soft-Tissue Calcifications

- Just as the location of a lesion is suggestive of its origin, calcifications visualized in periapical, panoramic, and CBCT images correlate with various soft-tissue calcifications.
- The most effective manner in which to diagnose them is to note the following:
  – Location.
  – Number.
    ○ Single.
    ○ Multiple.
  – Appearance.
    ○ Smooth outline.
    ○ Irregular outline.
- Common soft-tissue calcification often seen in panoramic radiographs is/are carotid calcifications (atherosclerosis, carotid plaques) which are visualized at the area of the bifurcation of the common carotid artery in the region of cervical vertebrae C3 and C4 (▶ Fig. 6.14).

The panoramic radiograph in ▶ Fig. 6.15 demonstrates a larger calcified plaque on the patient's left side than right side. An incidental finding such as this should alert the prudent dental clinician to consider a referral to the patient's physician for further vascular work-up; it may indicate an increased risk for cerebrovascular accident (stroke).

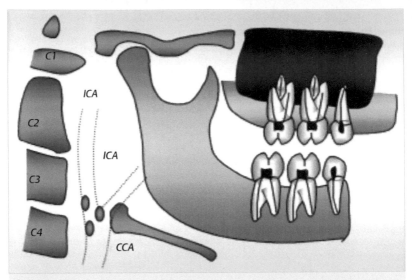

Fig. 6.14 Diagram demonstrating important hard and soft tissue anatomic landmarks that can be seen in panoramic radiographs. CCA, common carotid artery; ICA, internal carotid artery.

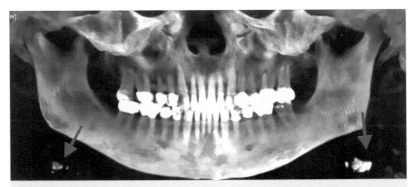

Fig. 6.15 Panoramic radiograph demonstrating bilateral carotid calcifications. The patient's left side demonstrates a larger calcified plaque than the right.

▶ Fig. 6.16 shows a panoramic radiograph with bilateral multiple small radiopacities in the mandibular third molar/ramus area. This is a common location and appearance for palatine tonsil calcifications (tonsilloliths).

100

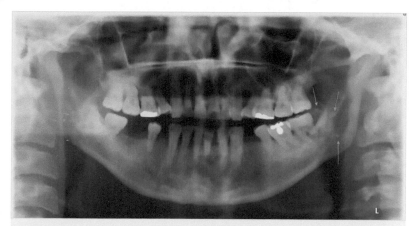

Fig. 6.16 Panoramic radiograph demonstrating bilateral multiple small tonsilloliths (denoted by the *blue arrows*).

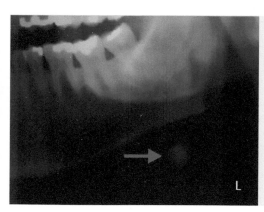

Fig. 6.17 Section of a panoramic radiograph demonstrating a left submandibular sialolith, a calcification within the submandibular gland.

In the portion of the panoramic image shown in ▶ Fig. 6.17, the single well-defined radiopacity in the soft tissue area inferior to the left angle of the mandible is most consistent with a submandibular gland calcification (submandibular sialolith), which is a calcification within the submandibular gland.

In the occlusal image of ▶ Fig. 6.18, note the well-defined elongated radiopacity in the left submandibular (Wharton) duct. This is an example of a submandibular sialolith.

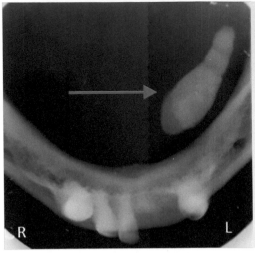

Fig. 6.18 Occlusal radiograph demonstrating a well-defined elongated radiopacity in the left submandibular (Wharton) duct. This is a submandibular sialolith.

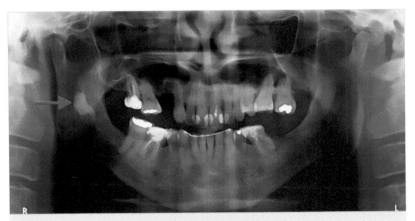

Fig. 6.19 Panoramic radiograph demonstrating a well-defined homogeneous radiopacity in the area of the right parotid gland. This suggests a parotid sialolith.

► Fig. 6.19 shows a panoramic radiograph demonstrating a well-defined homogeneous radiopacity in the area of the right parotid gland and beginning of the parotid duct. This calcification is suggestive of a parotid gland sialolith.

► Fig. 6.20 shows a panoramic radiograph demonstrating calcified stylo-hyoid complexes on both the right and left sides.

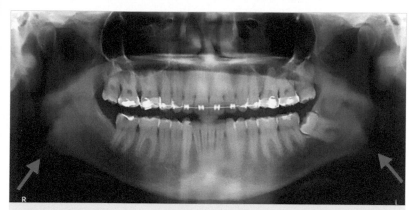

Fig. 6.20 Panoramic radiograph demonstrating bilateral calcified stylohyoid complexes.

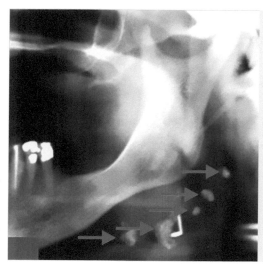

Fig. 6.21 Cropped panoramic radiograph demonstrating multiple lymph node calcifications in the soft tissue below the inferior border of the left angle.

In the cropped panoramic radiographic image above (▶ Fig. 6.21), the multiple bead-like radiopacities in the soft tissue below the inferior border of the left angle of the mandible are consistent with lymph node calcifications. There are several areas in the head and neck where lymph nodes may appear in radiography (▶ Fig. 6.22). A lymph node calcification may also resemble a large cauliflower-like radiopacity below the inferior aspect of the mandible.

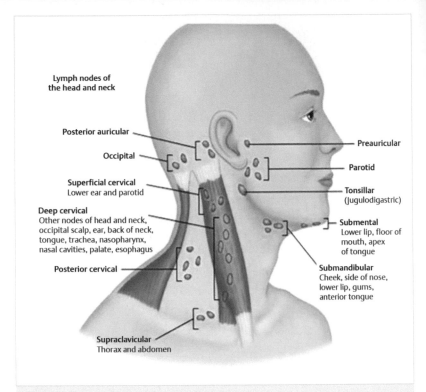

Lymph nodes of the head and neck

Posterior auricular

Occipital

Superficial cervical
Lower ear and parotid

Deep cervical
Other nodes of head and neck,
occipital scalp, ear, back of neck,
tongue, trachea, nasopharynx,
nasal cavities, palate, esophagus

Posterior cervical

Supraclavicular
Thorax and abdomen

Preauricular

Parotid

Tonsillar
(Jugulodigastric)

Submental
Lower lip, floor of
mouth, apex
of tongue

Submandibular
Cheek, side of nose,
lower lip, gums,
anterior tongue

Fig. 6.22 Diagram demonstrating the various areas in the head and neck region where lymph nodes may appear in radiography.

On the right side in the panoramic radiograph shown in ▶ Fig. 6.23, notice the multiple well-defined radiopacities with radiolucencies in the center (bulls-eye appearance), which is the common appearance of a phlebolith. Phleboliths are idiopathic calcifications (or calcinoses) that result from deposition of calcium in the normal tissue.

▶ Fig. 6.24 demonstrates a panoramic radiograph where a single well-defined radiopacity is seen in the area of the right nasal cavity. This entity is highly suggestive of a rhinolith (calcification in the nasal cavity).

▶ Fig. 6.25 demonstrates a periapical radiograph that shows a small well-defined radiopacity within the boundaries of the right maxillary sinus. This is suggestive of a calcification in the sinus, which is called an antrolith. Dystrophic calcification in the sinuses can also be seen in cases of chronic sinusitis or fungal sinusitis.

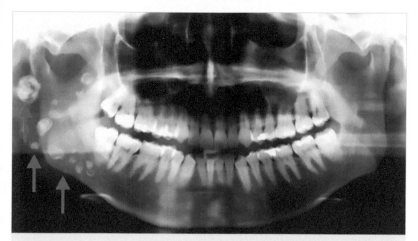

Fig. 6.23 Panoramic radiograph demonstrating multiple well-defined radiopacities with radiolucencies in the center (bull's eye)—the common appearance of phleboliths.

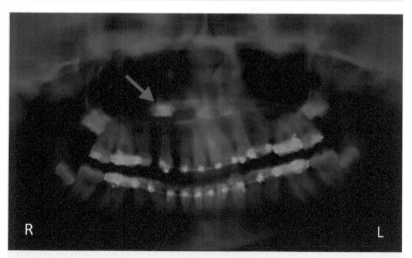

Fig. 6.24 Panoramic radiograph demonstrating a single well-defined radiopacity in the area of the right nasal cavity—suggestive of a rhinolith.

▶ Fig. 6.26 shows a coronal CBCT image demonstrating the presence of multiple small well-defined radiopacities along the floor of the right maxillary sinus. These are also suggestive of antroliths.

105

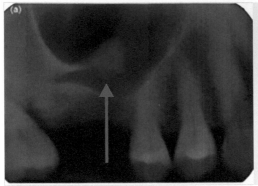

Fig. 6.25 Periapical radiograph demonstrating a small well-defined radiopacity within the boundaries of the right maxillary sinus—consistent with antrolith.

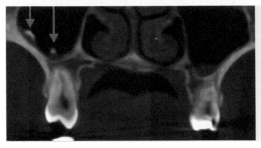

Fig. 6.26 Coronal cone beam computed tomography image demonstrating multiple small well-defined radiopacities along the floor of the right maxillary sinus—suggestive of antroliths.

One of the most common types of mandibular radiopacities are islands of dense cortical bone within the boundaries of the buccal and lingual cortical plates. These are called *dense bone islands*, or *idiopathic osteosclerosis*, or *enostosis*. This phenomenon is a self-limiting condition of bone and does not require further evaluation or treatment. On rare occasions, they may cause root resorption or may make orthodontic tooth movement more difficult.

▶ Fig. 6.27 shows a panoramic radiograph demonstrating a well-defined radiopacity with no lucent rim/border in the right body of the mandible near the apices of the right mandibular second premolar/right mandibular first molar (teeth #29 and 30). Enostoses are usually painless and typically do not cause swelling, pain, or changes in nerve sensation.

▶ Fig. 6.28 shows a cross-sectional view from a CBCT of two separate enostoses/dense bone islands/idiopathic osteoscleroses—one is more inferiorly positioned to the other. Note the "lesions" extend from the buccal to the lingual cortices and do not have a lucent rim, nor do they cause cortical expansion.

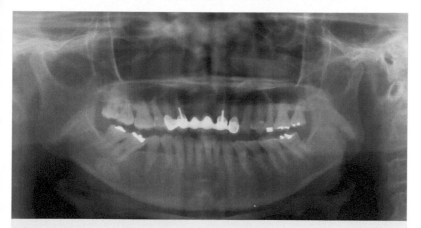

Fig. 6.27 Panoramic radiograph demonstrating a well-defined radiopacity with no lucent rim in the right body of the mandible—consistent with enostosis.

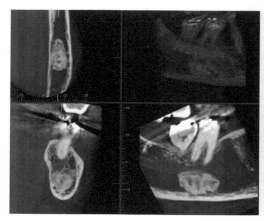

Fig. 6.28 Multi- and cross-sectional cone beam computed tomography views of the enostosis seen in ▶ Fig. 6.27 that demonstrate a dense bone island/enostosis that nearly spans the entire width of the body of the mandible.

▶ Fig. 6.29 shows the different types of dense bone island/enostosis/idiopathic osteosclerosis presentations within the cortical (buccal or lingual) plates. In each of the images, the left side represents the buccal cortex, while the right side represents the lingual. Note the various pattern possibilities for these very common "lesions."

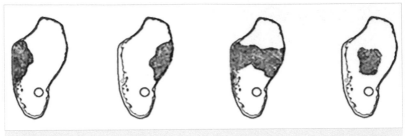

Fig. 6.29 Diagram showing the different types of enostosis pattern presentations within the cortical plates.

It is important to understand that the entities discussed in this chapter represent only some of the most common presentations of those conditions. The same entities may have different radiographic appearances, or a similar-appearing abnormality may be a totally different pathology that requires clinical attention. It may also be prudent to consider consulting a specialist when doubt remains about the diagnoses at hand.

7 Odontogenic Infections

Chan M. Park, Benjamin R. Shimel, Jeffrey A. Elo, Alan S. Herford

Introduction

- One of the more difficult problems to manage in dentistry.
- Commonly arise from the teeth and have characteristic flora.
- Caries and periodontal disease lead to pulpitis and apical periodontitis that can spread to the alveolar process as well as the deeper tissues of the face, oral cavity, head, and neck.
- Infections vary in severity.
- May range from low-grade, well-localized infections that require only minimal treatment to severe, life-threatening deep fascial space infections.
- Although the majority of infections are managed by minor surgical procedures and antibiotic administration, sometimes these infections can occasionally become severe and life-threatening in a short time.

Microbiology of Odontogenic Infections

- Causative bacteria that are part of the normal oral flora include:
  - Bacteria from plaque.
  - Mucosal surface organisms.
  - Gingival sulcus flora.
- Progression of bacterial species over time:
  - Aerobic gram-positive cocci.
    - Anaerobic gram-positive cocci.
      - Anaerobic gram-negative rods.
- These cause a variety of common diseases such as:
  - Dental caries.
  - Gingivitis.
  - Periodontitis.

Microflora Activity

- When the bacteria gain access to deeper tissues, such as a necrotic dental pulp or a deep periodontal pocket, they can cause odontogenic infections.
- As the infection progresses deeper, different members of the infecting flora may find better growth conditions and outnumber the previously dominant species.
- Each infectious disease process is unique and differs according to:
  - Its anatomic location.
  - Etiologic microorganisms.

– Virulence patterns.
– Accessibility to surgical drainage.
– Signs and symptoms.
– Host response to the process.
• Orofacial infections are unique and do not mimic infections in other locations. These may be:
  – Chronic (e.g., periodontitis).
  – Chronic–subacute with acute exacerbations (e.g., pericoronitis, periodontal abscess).
  – Intensely acute (necrotizing ulcerative gingivitis, cellulitis with or without extension into the orbital or submandibular spaces).
  – Peri-implantitis.
  – Osteomyelitis.
  – Deep neck and fascial space infections.
  – Ludwig's angina.
  – Mediastinal infections.
  – Necrotizing fasciitis.
  – Cervicofacial actinomycosis.

Polymicrobial

• Almost all odontogenic infections are caused by multiple bacterial species.
• Laboratory results can typically identify an average of five species of bacteria.

Aerobic Versus Anaerobic

• An important factor is oxygen tolerance of the bacterial species.
• Aerobic bacteria alone account for 6% of all odontogenic infections.
• Anaerobic bacteria alone are the reason for 44% of odontogenic infections.
• Infections caused by a mixed population of anaerobic and aerobic bacteria comprise 50% of all odontogenic infections.

Aerobes

• The predominant aerobes (65% of cases) belong to the *Streptococcus milleri* group:
  – *S. anginosus.*
  – *S. intermedius.*
  – *S. constellatus.*
• These facultative organisms, which can grow in the presence or absence of oxygen, may also initiate spread into the deeper tissue layers.

Anaerobes

- Anaerobic gram-positive cocci are found in about 65% of cases.
- These cocci usually belong to the anaerobic *Streptococcus* and *Peptostreptococcus* species.

Pathophysiology of Odontogenic Infections

- The mechanism by which mixed aerobic and anaerobic bacteria cause infections has been established.
- After initial inoculation into the deeper tissues, the facultative *S. milleri* organisms can synthesize hyaluronidase which allows them to spread through connective tissues and initiate a cellulitis type of infection.
- Metabolic by-products from the *streptococci* then create a favorable environment for the growth of anaerobes.
  - The release of essential nutrients.
  - Lowered pH in the tissues.
  - Consumption of local oxygen supplies.
- As collagen is broken down and invading white blood cells necrose and lyse, microabscesses form and may coalesce into a clinically recognizable abscess.
- In the abscess stage, the anaerobic bacteria predominate and may eventually become the only organisms found in culture.
- Early infections (cellulitis) may be characterized as aerobic *streptococcal* infections; and late, chronic infections (abscess) may be characterized as anaerobic infections.
- Clinically, this progression from aerobic to anaerobic seems to correlate with the swelling that can be found in the infected region.
- Odontogenic infections pass through four stages:
- During the first 3 days, a soft, mildly tender, doughy swelling represents the *inoculation stage*, in which the invading *streptococci* are just beginning to colonize the host.
- After 3 to 5 days, the swelling becomes warm, hard, red, and acutely tender as the infecting mixed flora stimulates the intense inflammatory response of the *cellulitis stage*.
- At 5 to 7 days, the anaerobes begin to predominate, causing a liquefied abscess in the center of the swollen area. This is the *abscess stage*.
- Finally, when the abscess drains through skin or mucosa or it is surgically drained, the *resolution stage* begins as the immune system destroys the infecting bacteria and the processes of healing and repair ensue (▶ Table 7.1).

Table 7.1 Comparison of edema, cellulitis, and abscess

Characteristic	Edema (inoculation)	Cellulitis	Abscess
Duration	0–3 days	1–5 days	4–10 days
Pain, borders	Mild, diffuse	Diffuse	Localized
Size	Variable	Large	Smaller
Color	Normal	Red	Shiny center
Consistency	Jelly-like	Board-like	Soft center
Progression	Increasing	Increasing	Decreasing
Pus	Absent	Absent	Present
Bacteria	Aerobic	Mixed	Anaerobic
Seriousness	Low	Greater	Less

Origins of Odontogenic Infections

- Two major origins:
  - Periapical:
    - Results from pulpal necrosis and subsequent bacterial invasion into the periapical tissue.
  - Periodontal:
    - Results from deep periodontal pocketing that allows inoculation of bacteria into the underlying soft tissues.
- Of these two, the periapical origin is more common.

Spread of Infection

- The infection spreads through the cancellous bone until it encounters a cortical plate.
- If this cortical plate is thin, the infection may erode through the bone and enter the surrounding soft tissues.
- Treatment of the necrotic pulp by standard endodontic therapy or extraction of the tooth typically resolves the infection.
- Antibiotics alone may arrest the infection but usually fail at pathogen eradication because the underlying dental cause has not yet been treated.
- If the infection erodes through the cortical plate of the alveolar process, it spreads into predictable anatomic locations.

- The location of the infection arising from a specific tooth is determined by two major factors:
  - The thickness of the bone overlying the apex of the tooth.
  - The relationship of the site of perforation of bone to muscle attachments of the maxilla and mandible.
- Infection typically erodes into the soft tissue through the thinnest portions of cortical bone (path of least resistance):
  - If the root apex is near the thin labial bone, the infection erodes labially.
  - If the root apex is near the palatal aspect, the palatal bone will be perforated.

Muscle Attachments

- The location of bony perforation relative to muscle attachment determines the fascial space involved.
  - If the tooth apex is inferior to the muscle attachment sites, it results in a vestibular abscess.
  - If tooth apex is superior to the muscle attachments, adjacent fascial space involvement occurs.

Fascial Spaces Involved in Odontogenic Infections (▶ Table 7.2)

- Fascial spaces are potential spaces that exist between anatomic barriers which can be expanded into areas of edema in the presence of infection.
- Primary maxillary spaces are:
  - Canine.
  - Buccal.
  - Infratemporal.
- Primary mandibular spaces are:
  - Submental.
  - Buccal.
  - Submandibular.
  - Sublingual.
- Secondary fascial spaces are:
  - Masseteric.
  - Pterygomandibular.
  - Superficial and deep temporal.
  - Lateral pharyngeal.
  - Retropharyngeal.
  - Prevertebral.

Table 7.2 Fascial spaces and planes

Space	Odontogenic sources of infection	Contents of space
Buccal	Mandibular premolars Maxillary molars and premolars	- Parotid duct - Anterior facial artery/vein - Transverse facial artery/vein - Buccal fat pad
Infraorbital	Maxillary canine	- Angular artery/vein - Infraorbital nerve
Submandibular	Mandibular molars	- Submandibular gland - Facial artery/vein - Lymph nodes
Submental	Mandibular anteriors	- Anterior jugular vein - Lymph nodes
Sublingual	Mandibular molars and premolars	- Sublingual glands - Wharton's duct - Lingual nerve and artery - Sublingual artery/vein
Infratemporal	Maxillary molars	- Pterygoid plexus - Cranial nerve V3 (mandibular)

Abscess

- The most common location for an odontogenic deep fascial space abscess is the vestibular space.
- Presence of pus equates to abscess formation.
- An abscess indicates that the body has locally contained the infection and that the host resistance mechanisms have stabilized the infectious processes.
- An acute abscess is a more mature infection with more localized pain, decreased swelling, and well-circumscribed borders.
- The abscess is fluctuant on palpation because it is a pus-filled tissue pocket containing necrotic tissue, bacterial colonies, and dead white blood cells.
- A chronic abscess is usually slow-growing and less threatening than a cellulitis, especially if it has drained spontaneously to the external environment.
- Classically described as a localized, well-circumscribed fluctuant pocket containing necrotic tissue, anaerobic bacteria, and dead white blood cells (pus).
- Treatment is incision and drainage, along with definitive treatment of the offending tooth.

Cellulitis

- An acute, painful infection with increased swelling and diffuse borders.
- Maintains a firm consistency upon palpation and contains no pus.

- May be a rapidly spreading process in serious infections.
- Classically described as a warm, diffuse, erythematous, indurated, and painful swelling of the tissues in an infected area.
- Treatment is antibiotics, with possible incision and drainage if there is no improvement over 2 to 3 days, or if there is evidence of purulence (pus) or risk of airway compromise.

Orofacial Infections (other types)

- Cavernous sinus thrombosis:
  - Spread of an odontogenic infection from the maxilla to the cavernous sinus is via a hematogenous route.
  - The veins of the head and orbit lack valves, so this process can occur via one of two potential routes:
    - Inferiorly via alveolar veins to the pterygoid plexus to the emissary veins.
    - Superiorly via the angular vein and the superior or inferior ophthalmic veins.
- Ludwig's angina:
  - It is a bilateral infection of the submandibular space that consists of two compartments in the floor of the mouth: the sublingual space and the submylohyoid (also known as submaxillary) space.
  - The infection is a rapidly spreading cellulitis without lymphatic involvement and generally without abscess formation.
  - This leads to difficulty swallowing or breathing and is considered a true emergency.

Osteoradionecrosis (ORN)

- Radiation of the head and neck results in permanent damage to bone and osteocytes as well as the microvasculature.
- The radiated/altered bone becomes hypoxic, hypovascular, and hypocellular.
- This altered bone is broken down and a nonhealing wound develops in which the tissues' metabolic demand exceeds its supply.
- Most cases arise secondary to local trauma after radiation.
- ORN can also occur spontaneously following radiation.
- ORN most frequently affects the mandible.
- Clinical presentation of ORN:
  - Diagnosis of ORN requires at least 3 to 5 mm of intraoral exposed bone in an irradiated field that is present for at least 6 months.
  - Other clinical features include:
    - Intractable pain.
    - Cortical perforation.
    - Fistula formation.
    - Surface ulceration
    - Pathologic fracture.

- Radiographic presentation of ORN:
  - Ill-defined zone of radiolucency that may develop zones of relative radiopacity.
- Prevention of ORN:
  - Extractions should occur prior to radiation with at least 3 weeks healing time (prior to the initiation of radiation) or within 4 months post radiation.
  - Procedures following the 4th month (*golden period*) should be preceded and followed by hyperbaric oxygen therapy.

Medication-Related Osteonecrosis of the Jaws (MRONJ)

- Reports of osteonecrosis of the jaws in patients taking intravenous bisphosphonates zoledronic acid (Zometa®) and pamidronic acid (Aredia®) in high doses for metastatic cancers or multiple myeloma began to arise in 2003.
- The majority of cases have been associated with dental procedures such as tooth extraction.
- MRONJ also occurs spontaneously without any inciting (traumatic) event.
- Cases of MRONJ have also been associated with the use of oral bisphosphonates alendronic acid (Fosamax®), risedronic acid (Actonel®), and ibandronic acid (Boniva®).
- The risk of MRONJ with oral bisphosphonate use is lower than the risk with intravenous bisphosphonate use.
- Clinical presentation of MRONJ:
  - Generally presents with painful bone exposure.
  - Patients may also be asymptomatic with the only significant finding being exposed (necrotic) bone.
  - Possible associated findings include:
    - Soft tissue edema (swelling).
    - Infection.
    - Loosening of teeth.
    - Drainage—often at the site of tooth extraction.
- Prevention of MRONJ:
  - Oral bisphosphonates
    - The American Dental Association recommends emphasis on conservative surgical techniques, proper sterile technique, and antibiotic therapy.
    - If the patient has been taking oral bisphosphonates for longer than 5 years, they may no longer benefit the patient; consultation with the patient's primary care provider may be advised.
  - Intravenous bisphosphonates
    - Dental procedures should be avoided if at all possible while the patient is undergoing intravenous therapy; especially after 3 months of therapy.

Chronic Infection

- Sinus tract or fistula is often present.
- Occasionally, patients do not seek treatment for these infections and the process ruptures spontaneously and drains, occasionally resulting in resolution but typically leading to chronicity of the infection.
- The infection recurs if the site of spontaneous drainage becomes occluded.
- Sometimes the abscess establishes a chronic sinus tract that drains to the oral cavity or the skin.
- Chronic drainage sinus tracts that result from low-grade infections may drain intraorally or extraorally.
- As long as the sinus tract continues to drain, the patient has no pain.
- Antibiotics usually stop the pus drainage; but when the antibiotic course concludes, drainage recurs.
- Definitive treatment of a chronic sinus tract requires treatment of the original causative problem, which is usually a necrotic pulp (root canal treatment vs. extraction).

Principles of Therapy of Odontogenic Infections

- Determine severity of infection.
  - Most are mild and require only minor surgical therapy.
  - Take a good history:
    - Typical chief complaints: (e.g., "I have a toothache"; "My jaw is swollen" or "I have a bump in my gums")
    - Determine how long the infection has been present (e.g., "When did it start?" or "Any drainage, pain, redness?")
  - Elicit the patient's symptoms.
  - Infections are often severe inflammatory responses and the cardinal signs of inflammation are easy to discern clinically.
    - *Dolor* (pain).
    - *Tumor* (swelling).
    - *Calor* (warmth).
    - *Rubor* (erythema, redness).
    - *Functio laesa* (loss of function).
- Pain:
  - The most common complaint is *dolor* (pain).
    - Where the pain actually started.
    - "How has the pain spread since it was first noted?"
- Swelling:
  - The second sign is *tumor* (swelling).
  - Swelling is a physical finding that is sometimes subtle and not obvious to the practitioner, although it is obvious to the patient.

117

- Warmth:
  - The third characteristic of infection is *calor* (warmth).
    - "Has the area felt warm to the touch?"
- Redness:
  - *Rubor* or redness of the overlying area.
    - "Has there been any change in color, especially redness, over the area of the infection?"
- Loss of function:
  - Loss of function should be ruled out.
    - "Do you have difficulty opening your mouth (*trismus*) widely?"
    - Is it difficult to chew, swallow (*dysphagia*), or breathe (*dyspnea*)?
- Malaise:
  - Patients who feel fatigued, feverish, weak, and sick are said to have *malaise*.
  - Malaise usually indicates a generalized reaction to a moderate or severe infection.
- Self-treatment:
  - Ask about previous professional treatment and self-treatment.
  - Many patients doctor themselves with leftover antibiotics, hot soaks, and a variety of other home or herbal remedies.

Physical Examination

- The first step in the physical examination is to obtain the patient's vital signs including:
  - Temperature.
  - Blood pressure.
  - Pulse rate.
  - Respiratory rate.
- These signs point to an immune response mounted by the body.
- Patients with severe odontogenic infections can present with elevated temperature, pulse rate, and respiratory rate.
- Temperature:
  - Patients who have systemic involvement of infection have temperatures elevated to 101 °F or higher (greater than 38.3 °C).
- Pulse:
  - Pulse rate increases as the patient's temperature increases.
  - Pulse rates of up to 100 beats/minute are common in patients with infections.
  - If pulse rates increase to greater than 100 beats/minute, consider a severe infection and treat more aggressively.
- Blood pressure:
  - The vital sign that varies the *least* with infections is blood pressure.
  - An elevation in systolic blood pressure occurs only if the patient has significant pain and/or anxiety.

- However, severe septic shock and profound infection results in hypotension.
- Respiratory rate:
  - The respiratory rate should be observed closely.
  - One major consideration is the potential for partial or complete upper airway obstruction as a result of the infection extending into the deep fascial spaces of the neck.
  - Normal respiratory rate is 10 to 16 breaths per minute.
  - Patients with mild to moderate infections may have elevated respiratory rates at greater than 18 breaths per minute.

Management

- Patients who have abnormal vital signs with elevation of temperature, pulse rate, and/or respiratory rate are more likely to have a serious infection and require more intensive therapy with evaluation by an oral and maxillofacial surgeon (OMS) or evaluation in the emergency room (ER).
- Review the medical history carefully for:
  - Diabetes.
  - Severe renal disease.
  - Alcoholism with malnutrition.
  - Leukemias and lymphomas.
  - Cancer chemotherapy.
  - Immunosuppressive therapy of any kind.
- These comorbidities may result in less vital sign abnormalities than expected (an afebrile patient) despite systemic involvement of the infection due to immune suppression.
- An infection in these patients must be treated much more vigorously because the infection may spread more rapidly.
- Referral to an OMS must be considered for early, aggressive surgery to remove the cause and to initiate intensive parenteral (IV) antibiotic therapy.

Criteria for Referral to an OMS or the Emergency Room

- Difficulty breathing (*dyspnea*).
- Difficulty swallowing (*dysphagia*).
- Dehydration.
- Moderate to severe trismus (interincisal opening less than 20 mm).
- Swelling extending beyond the alveolar process.
- Elevated temperature (greater than 101°F).
- Severe malaise and toxic appearance.
- Compromised host defenses.
- Need for general anesthesia.
- Failed prior treatment.

Treat Infection Surgically

- For a typical infection, the most likely appearance is a carious tooth with a periapical radiolucency and a small vestibular abscess.
- The *primary* method for treating infections is to perform surgery to remove the source of the infection and, if necessary, to drain the anatomic spaces affected by the indurated cellulitis or abscess.
  - Root canal therapy.
  - Extraction, with or without incision and drainage.
- Indications for incision and drainage for abscessed lesions:
  - Antibiotics do not diffuse well into infected (pus-filled) areas.
  - Some antibiotics are inactive at abscesses (acidic pH).
  - Abscess microorganisms may not be replicating or metabolizing, negating the effects of antibiotics which require active intracellular molecular pathways for proper function (particularly beta-lactams such as penicillins and cephalosporins).
  - High levels of antibiotic inhibitors (e.g., beta-lactamases or other enzymes) may be present to inactivate the antibiotics.
  - Incision and drainage can induce postsurgical healing and angiogenesis to cause a high degree of vascularization in an area that now has a significantly reduced volume of infectious pathogens.
  - Increased vascularization indicates faster delivery of antibiotics to an area that now also hosts fewer microorganisms.
- To incise and drain:
  - Abscess is incised with a No. 11 or No. 15 scalpel blade.
  - Beaks of a hemostat are inserted through the incision and opened so that the disengaged beaks break up any loculations of pus.
  - Never close hemostat beaks inside of an incision to avoid damaging deep structures.
  - The abscess cavity is irrigated with at least 50 mL of saline to dilute the microorganisms and remove the pus.
    - Once the irrigant returns clear from being in the abscess cavity, it can be reasonably assured that the pus has been removed—"The solution to pollution is dilution."
  - One or more small drains are inserted to the depths of the abscess cavity to discourage additional accumulation of pus.
    - Failure to do so will result in worsening of the infection and failure of the infection to resolve, even if antibiotics are given.
    - The drain is sutured into place with 1 or 2 nondissolvable sutures (3–0 silk or nylon).
- If the tooth cannot be salvaged or restored, it should be extracted as soon as possible.
  - A prior period of antibiotic therapy is not necessary.

- Contrary to widely held opinion, extraction of a tooth in the presence of infection does not promote the spread of infection.
- Several studies have shown that removal of a tooth in the presence of infection hastens its resolution and minimizes the complications of the infection such as time out of work, hospitalization, and the need for extraoral incision and drainage.
- If the tooth is not to be extracted, its pulp should be removed, which results in elimination of the cause and limited drainage through the apical foramen.
- Even if the tooth cannot be opened or extracted, an incision and drainage should be conducted.
- However, when the appropriate surgery cannot be immediately performed, antibiotics may be useful to slow the progression of infection.

Pericoronitis

- Mild condition that does not require antibiotics.
- However, if patient develops trismus, extraoral swelling, and/or fever, irrigation and removal of the third molar/s will require supplementation with administration of antibiotics.
- Useful antibiotics are:
  - Penicillin.
  - Cephalexin.
  - Clindamycin.
  - Clarithromycin.

Indications for Therapeutic Use of Antibiotics

- Acute onset infection.
- Swelling extending beyond the alveolar process.
  - Diffuse swelling or involvement of fascial spaces.
- Cellulitis.
- Trismus.
- Lymphadenopathy.
- Temperature higher than 101°F.
- *Severe* pericoronitis.
- Osteomyelitis.
- Compromised host defenses.

Indications when Antibiotics are NOT Necessary

- Patient demand.
- Toothache.
- Well-localized periapical abscess.
- Minor vestibular abscess.

- Dry socket.
- Multiple dental extractions in a *non*-immunocompromised patient.
- Mild pericoronitis (inflammation of the operculum only).
- Drained alveolar abscess.
- Root canal sterilization.

Empiric Antibiotic Therapy

- The orally administered antibiotics that are effective against odontogenic infections include:
  - Penicillin.
  - Amoxicillin.
  - Clindamycin.
  - Azithromycin.
  - Metronidazole.
  - Moxifloxacin.
- Narrow-spectrum antibiotics useful for *simple* odontogenic infections are:
  - Penicillin 250 to 500 mg (adults).
    - #28 tabs, 1 tab PO (*by mouth*) qid (*four times daily*) until gone.
  - Clindamycin 150 mg (adults).
    - #28 caps, 1 cap PO qid until gone.
  - Metronidazole 500 mg (adults).
    - #21 tabs, 1 tab PO tid (*three times daily*) until gone.
- Broad-spectrum antibiotics useful for *complex* odontogenic infections are:
  - Amoxicillin 500 mg (adults).
    - #21 caps, 1 cap PO tid until gone.
  - Amoxicillin with clavulanic acid—for concurrent sinus infections.
    - 500 mg tabs, #30 tabs, 1 tab PO tid until gone; or
    - 875 mg tabs, #20 tabs, 1 tab PO bid (*twice daily*) until gone.
  - Azithromycin
    - 250 mg tabs, #6 tabs, 2 tabs PO as a single dose on day 1, followed by 250 mg PO daily until gone.
  - Tetracycline 500 mg (adults)
    - #28 tabs, 1 tab PO qid until gone.
  - Moxifloxacin 400 mg (adults).
    - #7 tabs, 1 tab PO daily until gone.
- Use bacteri*cidal*, if possible, rather than bacterio*static* antibiotics (penicillin is better than azithromycin) especially with immunocompromised patients.

Bibliography

[1] Hupp JR, Ellis E III, Tucker MR. Contemporary Oral and Maxillofacial Surgery, 6th ed. St. Louis, MO: Elsevier Mosby; 2014

8 Dentoalveolar Surgery

Christopher F. Viozzi, Jeffrey A. Elo

Indications for Tooth Extraction

- Severe caries (nonrestorable tooth).
- Pulpal necrosis/irreversible pulpitis.
  - Root canal therapy failure.
  - Tooth not a candidate for endodontic treatment.
- Severe periodontal disease.
- Combined endodontic-periodontic lesion.
- Tooth malposition/eruption disturbances due to:
  - Impaction.
  - Crowded arch.
  - Overeruption.
- Supernumerary teeth:
  - The mesiodens is the most common supernumerary tooth.
- Teeth associated with pathology.
- Fractured tooth (nonrestorable): Vertical root fracture.
- Pre-prosthetic extractions.
- Orthodontic indications.
- Medical indications:
  - Preradiation therapy (XRT)
  - Precardiac surgery (valve replacement or valve repair)
  - Pretransplant surgery
  - Pre-bisphosphonate therapy (especially IV bisphosphonates)

Contraindications (Relative) for Elective Tooth Extraction

- Systemic:
  - Uncontrolled diabetes:
    - Leukocyte dysfunction and decreased chemotaxis and phagocytosis occur when blood glucose is > 250 mg/dL (HbA$_{1c}$ > 10%)
  - End-stage renal disease with severe uremia.
  - Uncontrolled leukemia or lymphoma.
  - Uncontrolled cardiac disease:
    - Uncontrolled hypertension.
    - Unstable angina.
    - Recent myocardial infarction (MI).

- Severe bleeding disorders:
  - Hemophilia.
  - Thrombocytopenia (low platelet count).
- Pregnancy:
  - First and third trimester.
- Patients taking certain medications:
  - IV bisphosphonates.
  - Chemotherapeutic agents.
  - Anticoagulants.
  - Steroids.
- Local factors:
  - History of radiation therapy to the jaws (XRT).
  - Teeth within a tumor.
  - Severe pericoronitis with limited success at local anesthesia.

Extraction Procedure—Nonsurgical Extraction

Preparation—Preoperative Considerations

- Patient's health/medical history:
  - How will you manage medical comorbidities perioperatively?
  - Current medications and allergies.
  - Potential complications and how to best treat those conditions.
  - Current and signed treatment plan and consent form/s.
  - Initial blood pressure reading should be less than 160/100 for elective dental treatment (see Chapter 12, Hypertension Guidelines).
  - Your approach to the treatment:
    - Local anesthetic: which will you use?
    - Instruments: do you have what you need?
    - Aseptic technique (*in chronologic order*): wear mask and protective eyewear and surgical gown, wash hands, don gloves and avoid contact with nonsurgical surfaces.
    - Mentally reiterate and describe the extraction process.
    - Postop prescription options (see Chapter 15, Prescription Writing).

Presentation

- Depending on the setting (e.g., dental school clinic), the provider may be expected to give a brief verbal presentation to a supervising faculty on the proposed extraction.
- Typically, this presentation includes the following components:
  - Patient's pertinent medical history: Listing and current status of medical conditions that may affect ability to provide dental treatment.

- Current medications.
- Allergies.
- Surgical needs.
- Name any potential complications and how to manage any of those conditions in the surgical setting.
- Perform time out procedure (see Chapter 3, Time Out Policy: Correct Patient, Correct Procedure, Correct Site).
  - This helps ensure the correct patient, correct procedure, and correct site.

Clinical Attire

- Scrubs or business attire when working in the clinical setting.
- Long hair should be pulled back and secured (rubber bands, hair net/covering, etc.).
- Facial hair should be well kept and trimmed.
  - Perfume and cologne should not be worn (due to patient sensitivities/allergies).
- Jewelry should be left unworn:
  - No rings.
  - No dangling earrings.
- Open-toed shoes should be avoided.

Surgical Armamentarium

Proper surgical instrumentation is required to successfully complete simple or surgical extraction procedure. The practitioner must develop familiarity with the armamentarium to understand which instruments he/she prefers for each procedure, and then develop a standard tray with all of the desired instruments.

Each instrument, even those similar in appearance to others, serves a unique function; therefore, a well-developed, consistently arranged surgical tray provides a familiar workspace for greater ease with each planned procedure. This also helps prevent the practitioner from using an inappropriate instrument for something other than its planned purpose.

▶ Fig. 8.1 demonstrates a typical oral surgery tray set-up for either a simple or surgical extraction procedure. Items shown are named and described (*left to right, starting from the top row left*):
- Shaded lightweight protective glasses for the patient to wear.
  - Shaded glasses are important to give the patient's eyes some relief from the bright operatory lights and to prevent potential injury to the eyes when using surgical instruments.
- Tongue blade with petroleum jelly and a cotton tip applicator to apply the jelly to the patient's lips.
  - Provides comfort to the lips and helps prevent drying or cracking of the lips.

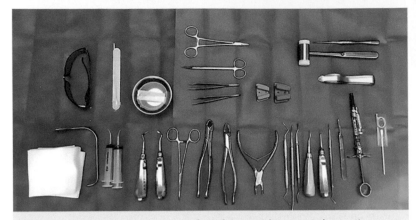

Fig. 8.1 Typical oral surgery tray set-up for either a simple or surgical extraction procedure.

- Stainless steel cup of normal saline (irrigant).
  - Placing the 3–0 chromic gut suture into the irrigant while the procedure is being performed allows the suture to soften and makes knot-tying easier.
- Needle holder (Mayo Hegar 6″): a holder used to grasp the suture needle while suturing.
- Scissors (Kelly Straight 6¼″): surgical scissors used to cut the suture knot.
- Adson-Brown tissue forceps: used for holding and manipulating delicate tissues.
- Adson tissue forceps: used to stabilize soft tissue for suturing, manipulation, or dissection.
- Child-sized bite block: firm block used to help assist patient in mouth opening.
- Adult-sized bite block: firm block used to help assist patient in mouth opening.
- Periotome (bayonet tip): gentle tapping facilitates atraumatic controlled extractions, especially of maxillary teeth.
- Mallet: used to gently tap periotome, facilitating atraumatic controlled extractions, especially of maxillary teeth.
- Minnesota retractor: an offset retractor used for the retraction of cheeks and soft-tissue flaps.
- Topical anesthetic (*shown is 20% benzocaine gel in a single-use package*): used on oral mucosa prior to local anesthesia injections.
- Dental injection syringe: a standard syringe used to administer local anesthetic.

- A #3 scalpel handle with a #15 blade attached: standard surgical blades dull quickly when they contact bone, teeth, or even with repeated use through soft tissue.
- Hirschfeld #20 periosteal elevator: a rounded elevator used primarily to reflect soft tissue once an incision has been made.
  - It is the preferred elevator for reflecting soft tissue because it has no sharp points and is unlikely to cause damage to the soft tissue or flap.
- Bayonet elevator: a specialized "lever" used to loosen teeth by stretching then severing the periodontal ligament attachments.
  - It has a sharp tip and a very thin but durable blade that may be helpful for use in tight contact areas.
- #77 R elevator: a specialized "lever" used to loosen teeth by stretching then severing the periodontal ligament attachments.
  - Possesses an offset blade with serrations to prevent slippage.
  - Difficult to use in tight contact areas.
- Double-ended bone file: used for smoothing small, sharp edges of bone.
- #9 periosteal elevator: a double-sided elevator that may be used to reflect soft tissue once an incision has been made. This can be accomplished through three methods:
  - Twisting or prying motion: the pointed end is used to reflect soft tissue, most commonly when elevating a dental papilla from between teeth or the attached gingiva around a tooth to be extracted.
  - Push stroke: the pointed or the broad end of the instrument is pushed underneath the periosteum, separating it from the underlying bone to produce a clean reflection.
  - Pull stroke: a withdrawing motion that tends to shred or tear the periosteum unless made carefully.
- Molt #2 angled double-ended (spoon) curette: used to remove granulation tissue from the extraction socket.
- Rongeur forceps: a grasping and cutting instrument used for removing bone.
- #150 Universal maxillary forceps: used to luxate and deliver maxillary teeth.
- #151 Universal mandibular forceps: used to luxate and deliver mandibular teeth.
- Hemostat (Kelly 5½"): a holder used to remove granulation tissue from the extraction socket and/or to pick up small debris (such as root tips, amalgam, or bone fragments).
- #190/191 elevators: a pair of specialized "levers" used to loosen teeth by stretching then severing the periodontal ligament attachments.
  - These are most often used for elevating maxillary third molars or maxillary and mandibular molar roots once they have been sectioned.
- 12 mL curved-tipped plastic syringe(s): used for procedural irrigation with normal saline.

- Weider tongue retractor (*sweetheart retractor*): a broad, heart-shaped retractor that is serrated on one side to firmly engage the tongue and retract it anteromedially.
- 4″ × 4″ gauze: soft, absorbent material often used as a throat pack/guard while performing the oral surgical procedure.
  - Smaller 2″ × 2″ gauzes are not preferred in oral surgery due to their small size, which prevents adequate screening and poses an aspiration risk (especially in anesthetized patients who may not feel the gauze's presence).
- (*Not shown, but recommended for use in surgery*) 3.0 mm modified Frazier stainless steel aspirator/suction (tip): an aspirator used for surgical suction.

Preparing the Patient—Patient Positioning

Postural comfort of both the patient and the provider is an important consideration when performing surgery. Most patients can tolerate lying relatively flat for the short duration of time it will take to perform the procedure. However, a small number of patients may require other considerations before being placed in a supine position, such as those with cardiopulmonary issues who experience a drowning sensation when reclined (e.g., congestive heart failure patients), patients with claustrophobia, or those with neck or back issues who experience pain.

For a typical oral surgery procedure, the patient should be placed horizontally on his/her back with the head elevated about 20 to 30 degrees—reminiscent of a "beach chair" position. A level, even surgical field allows for the greatest ease of movement for a focused practitioner. It is worth noting that with the patient in this position and with the mouth opened, the maxillary teeth are essentially perpendicular to the floor, and the mandibular teeth are parallel to the floor. This permits use of the surgical instrumentation to maximum advantage.

Another very important consideration is the height of the chair once the patient is reclined. To assert a relaxed and comfortable posture, the surgeon's elbows should remain comfortably at his/her sides at approximately 90 degrees (▶ Fig. 8.2).

A chair positioned too low may lead to lumbar or leg pain from strain, while a high chair could force a "shrugged" position and sore shoulders. Determining one's proper chair height is a trial-and-error process that is worthwhile before entering practice. Most dental chairs feature preset capabilities that allow them to "remember" a preferred height.

Patient Protection and Comfort Devices

The safety of the patient is the utmost priority, followed closely by patient comfort. To accomplish these goals, a hair net or surgical hair cover is recommended to keep the patient's own hair out of the surgical site. Shaded, protective eyewear can also keep the eyes protected from any instruments or irritants while preventing ocular irritation from the bright surgical lights overhead. A bite block should be placed to alleviate tension in the muscles and to allow the temporomandibular joints (TMJs) to relax while the procedure is being performed (▸ Fig. 8.3).

Lubricating or moisturizing products such as petroleum jelly should be applied to the patient's lips to coat all the skin surfaces, including the commissures, to prevent and protect against dryness and damage from desiccation (▸ Fig. 8.4). If the lips are not particularly dry, then delaying this until the procedure is complete may be preferable to avoid the inevitable transfer of lubricant from the patient to the practitioner, with the potential for loss of instrument control.

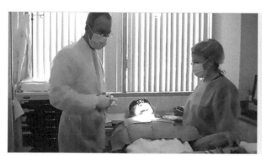

Fig. 8.2 To assert a relaxed and comfortable posture, the surgeon's elbows should remain comfortably at his/her sides at approximately 90 degrees.

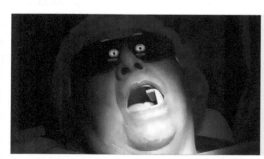

Fig. 8.3 Preparing the patient for surgery includes placement of a surgical hair cover, shaded protective eyewear, and a bite block.

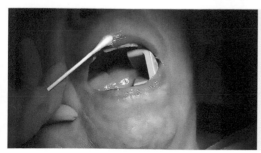

Fig. 8.4 Using a cotton tip applicator to apply petroleum jelly to the lips to help prevent dryness and cracking during the procedure.

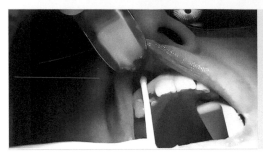

Fig. 8.5 A Minnesota retractor is used to gently retract the patient's lip to place the topical local anesthetic gel.

Obtain Profound Local Anesthesia—Topical Anesthesia

A Minnesota retractor is used to gently retract the patient's lip to place the topical local anesthetic gel (▶ Fig. 8.5).

The gel should be left in place for 60 seconds to exert an appropriate anesthetic response. Care should be taken to avoid retracting the lip so much as to cause (nasal) airway obstruction or to cause damage to the underlying vestibular mucosa, as the metal edge of the Minnesota retractor may cause abrasion or ulceration if placed too firmly against the epithelium.

Local Anesthetic Administration—Maxillary Infiltration

In the case shown in these photos, the maxillary right lateral incisor is to be extracted. The maxillary buccal infiltration, palatal infiltration, and periodontal ligament (PDL) or intragingival infiltration injections are recommended to achieve profound local anesthesia and chemical hemostasis that will allow for the most comfortable, painless, and bloodless procedure. Maxillary buccal infiltration (▶ Fig. 8.6) alone may provide profound pulpal and buccal soft-tissue anesthesia to most upper dentition, but will likely fall short of achieving complete, profound anesthesia for an extraction procedure.

Palatal Infiltration

Palatal infiltration (▶ Fig. 8.7) is necessary to anesthetize the palatal soft tissues and, in some cases, to achieve accessory pulpal anesthesia in 2-rooted maxillary premolars and 3-rooted maxillary molars. It is prudent to deliver this injection very slowly to avoid severe pain.

Periodontal Ligament or Intragingival Infiltration

PDL or intragingival infiltration (▶ Fig. 8.8) provides additional assurances for profound pulpal anesthesia while displacing capillary blood cells from the area—evidenced by blanching of the soft tissues—that can help reduce bleeding during extraction.

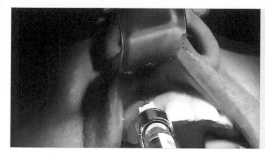

Fig. 8.6 Maxillary buccal infiltration to provide pulpal and buccal soft-tissue anesthesia.

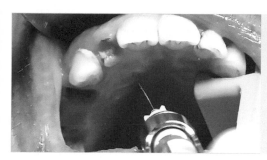

Fig. 8.7 Palatal infiltration is necessary to anesthetize the palatal soft tissues.

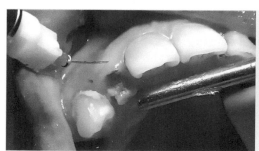

Fig. 8.8 Periodontal ligament or intragingival infiltration provides additional assurances for profound pulpal anesthesia while displacing capillary blood cells from the area that can help reduce bleeding.

Protecting the Airway—Placing the Throat Pack/Guard

A single 4″ × 4″ gauze (do not use 2″ × 2″ or 3″ × 3″ as they are too small) is unfolded and gently placed as a throat pack/guard to protect the patient's airway from extraction debris. This will prevent unnecessary aspiration or swallowing hazards. The throat pack/guard should be comfortably tucked and secured posterior to the surgical site to eliminate spaces for the extraction debris to fall into (▶ Fig. 8.9).

131

Confirming Profound Local Anesthesia

The surgeon may test for adequate local anesthesia by placing a surgical instrument in the sulcus of the tooth to be removed. The instrument should be used to gently elevate the soft tissues—as well as the tooth—as the surgeon inquires, "Do you feel any *pain* when I do this?" instead of asking, "Do you feel *anything* when I do this?" The inquiry must be specific about *pain* because the sensation of *pressure* is normally present even under proper anesthesia. If the patient affirms that they do *not* feel *pain*, but only feel *pressure*, remind them that *pressure* is normal. Should the patient feel *pain*, more anesthetic may be administered. Instruments such as the double-ended Molt #2 spoon-shaped curette (▶ Fig. 8.10), a #9 periosteal elevator, or the Hirschfeld periosteal elevator are appropriate for this confirmation test.

Each of these instruments can also be used to gently and circumferentially sever the crestal/sulcular dentogingival fibers.

Periotomes

For every erupted maxillary tooth requiring removal, the use of the periotome may be helpful. The dental assistant should facilitate the procedure by gently retracting the patient's cheek with a Minnesota retractor to allow good visibility and light. With his/her other hand, the dental assistant should keep

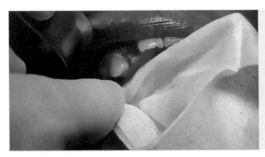

Fig. 8.9 The throat pack/ guard should be comfortably tucked and secured posterior to the surgical site to eliminate spaces for the extraction debris to fall into.

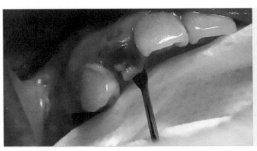

Fig. 8.10 The Molt #2 spoon-shaped curette is used to test for profound anesthesia while also gently severing the sulcular dentogingival fibers.

the suction tip around the sulcus of the tooth to be extracted to allow for a bloodless view of the operative site.

The surgeon should then place the tip of the periotome in the sulcus ensuring it is placed between the tooth (to be removed) and surrounding alveolar bone following the long axis of the tooth. Using a mallet with the other hand, the surgeon then *gently* taps the opposite end of the periotome, slowly advancing the working end of the periotome toward the tooth's apex (▶ Fig. 8.11). Care must be taken to ensure the tapping is *gently* performed, as patients can experience dizziness or headache if the tapping is too intense.

Gentle, circumferential tapping around the entire tooth slowly maneuvers the periotome apically so that the horizontal and oblique fibers of the periodontal ligament are severed, loosening the tooth in a rapid and atraumatic fashion. The patient may be told, "You will feel some tapping in the area—like a little woodpecker tapping on the tooth." This paints somewhat of a less threatening mental imagery for the patient who is often anxious and apprehensive at the sight and sounds of a mallet. Alternatively, the periotome can be "rocked" back and forth to gently advance it into the socket. A twisting motion can be used once engaged into the PDL space to disrupt the PDL fibers and luxate the tooth.

Elevators

Using a bayonet elevator (or a #301 small, straight elevator), the tooth to be extracted should carefully, slowly, and gently be elevated/luxated to further loosen it prior to placement of the forceps. The tooth should always be approached from the *facial* surface. It is never recommended to elevate a tooth from the lingual/palatal. The elevator may slip to cause significant and unnecessary soft-tissue damage, puncture wounds, or bleeding.

Insert the elevator into the mesial or distal periodontal ligament space with firm and controlled apical pressure. The elevator should follow the long axis of the tooth. The concave surface of the blade of the elevator should face the tooth that is to be extracted. The elevator is then slowly rotated in such a

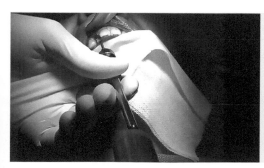

Fig. 8.11 Using a mallet, the surgeon gently taps the end of the periotome, slowly advancing the working end of the periotome toward the tooth's apex.

manner as to move the tooth toward the facial aspect. This is called *luxation* of the tooth. Care must be taken to avoid luxating adjacent teeth. Care must also be taken to avoid the use of elevators if they pose potential harm to adjacent teeth with large restorations or crowns.

Forceps Delivery

Following the circumferential use of the periotome around the tooth to its apex as well as luxation with the elevator, the #150 forceps (universal maxillary forceps) should be applied gently and carefully to the tooth to prevent pinching or tearing of the marginal gingiva (▶ Fig. 8.12).

A constant and firm apical pressure should be applied to the tooth using the forceps. This converts the center of rotation of the tooth from the apical third to the apex and helps to prevent root tip fractures. Take time to firmly establish the forceps position on the tooth as apically as possible. Using a combination of small circular movements, figure-8 movements, and a slight twisting motion (for teeth with a singular, conical root), the tooth may be delivered gently out of the socket. Take time while using the forceps to luxate and loosen the tooth. Allow the bone of the socket to expand rather than risk fracture from quick, uncontrolled movements. Once the tooth has been removed, place it onto the surgical tray table.

Care should also be taken to ensure that the gauze throat pack/guard remains in its proper place prior to tooth delivery in case any portion of the tooth cracks and fragments dislodge posteriorly. It is also critical for the dental assistant to use surgical suction/aspirators to provide a clear and bloodless view of the surgical site, helping ensure against notable tissue damage.

While individual preferences differ, an underhand grasp of the forceps (▶ Fig. 8.13) may be helpful in maintaining proper posture when extracting maxillary teeth.

This grasp encourages an ergonomic placement of the hands and wrists that keeps the elbows in a comfortable 90-degree angle and the spine in a straight posture. A natural vertebral positioning is also conducive to a relaxed stance of

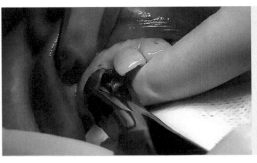

Fig. 8.12 The #150 forceps is applied gently and carefully to the tooth to prevent pinching or tearing of the marginal gingiva.

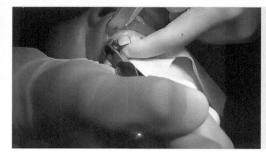

Fig. 8.13 An underhand grasp of the forceps may be helpful in maintaining proper posture when extracting maxillary teeth.

the shoulders. Note that the Minnesota retractor in the figure is *gently* reflecting the upper lip just enough to visualize the surgical site without obstructing the patient's nostrils and interfering with their ability to breathe comfortably.

Clinical Pearls

- Forceps selection options:
  - Maxillary universal (#150): can be used for all maxillary teeth.
  - Mandibular universal (#151): can be used for all mandibular teeth.
  - Cow horn (#23): can be used for mandibular molars with straight, minimally-curved roots.
    - Up and down (pump) motion works well with the #23 forceps.
  - Ash forceps: mandibular anterior teeth and premolars.
  - Maxillary molar anatomic forceps (#88 R and #88 L): can be used for maxillary molars with bifurcated or trifurcated, non-fused roots.

Clinical Pearls

- Tooth-specific forceps directional use:
  - Maxillary anterior teeth: rotate in the long axis of the tooth to be removed.
  - Maxillary premolars: luxate to the facial and palatal until there is a loss of resistance, then apply pulling pressure. This will help prevent root fracture. Often, first premolars are the only teeth to truly be "pulled."
  - Maxillary 1st and 2nd molars: facial and palatal luxation.
  - Maxillary 3rd molars: facial and distal luxation.
  - Mandibular anterior teeth and premolars: rotate in the long axis of the tooth.
  - Mandibular molars: when using the #23 forceps ("cow horn"), use a pump handle motion (up and down), then figure-8 motion, then roll out facially; when using the #151 forceps, use the figure-8 motion, then roll out facially.

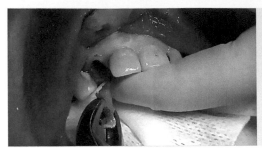

Fig. 8.14 Once the tooth has been delivered with the forceps, carefully inspect it to ensure that the complete tooth has been removed and that no root remnant remains.

Tooth Delivery

Once the tooth has been delivered with the forceps, carefully inspect it (▶ Fig. 8.14) to ensure that the complete tooth has been removed and that no root remnant remains.

Ensure a Clean and Smooth Socket

Examine and/or gently palpate the apical region of the socket to check for oral-antral communications (maxillary posterior teeth) and/or the presence of apical granulation/cyst tissue. Any periapical granulation/cystic tissue must be removed with a curette, and consideration should be given for submission of the tissue to an oral and maxillofacial pathologist for histopathologic examination and diagnosis.

Palpate the alveolar process on both the facial and lingual aspects of the socket to locate sharp bone edges and/or bony undercuts that could adversely affect the comfort of the patient. Finger palpation is usually adequate—if the ridge is sharp to finger palpation, it will certainly be sharp to the patient's tongue, lip, or buccal mucosa. If an area of sharpness is present, perform alveoloplasty—surgical contouring of the bone—with Rongeur forceps or a bone file.

Socket Irrigation

There is a saying in surgery that "*the solution to pollution is dilution.*" Most, if not all, infected surfaces are diluted thoroughly using a sterile solution to help reduce the prospect of bacteremia. Once the tooth has been removed, its socket is typically irrigated with 0.9% normal saline or sterile water. Gentle irrigation using a bulb syringe or a 12 mL curved plastic-tipped syringe (▶ Fig. 8.15) is best to access the small opening of the socket.

In the absence of pus, one syringe-full amount is sufficient to irrigate the extraction socket. If pus is present in the socket after tooth delivery, then 50 to

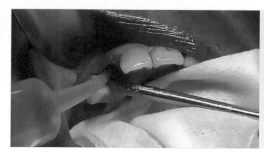

Fig. 8.15 Gentle irrigation of the socket using a 12 mL curved plastic-tipped syringe and normal saline or sterile water.

60 mL of irrigation is recommended to better dilute the infected site. Use of other irrigants in the presence of infection is not warranted (e.g., chlorhexidine, hydrogen peroxide, etc.) and can be injurious.

Suturing the Socket—Figure-8/Horizontal Mattress with Crossover Stitch

Evidence suggests that the incidence of dry socket—also known as alveolar osteitis—and postoperative infection can be reduced significantly in impacted mandibular third molar surgery with meticulous suture closure of the extraction site. This concept also holds true with single tooth or multiple teeth extraction sockets. Suturing over the socket encourages rapid healing by securing the marginal gingiva (which is responsible for epithelial migration across the socket), decreasing bleeding, securing osteitis-preventing clots, and reducing entrance of foreign debris to decrease the risk of infection.

For a single tooth extraction socket, a figure-8 (or horizontal mattress suture with crossover) is recommended. This suture provides a firm closure (or at least a minimization) of the socket opening while placing the suture knot on the facial surface of the gingiva, thereby limiting loosening interactions with the tongue so that the soft tissues are held firmly for an extended period of time (5–7 days).

This technique is initiated with the first pass made faciolingually through the distobuccal marginal gingiva toward its mesiopalatal counterpart (▶ Fig. 8.16).

Once through, the needle is then regrasped with the needle holder and passed first through the distopalatal marginal gingiva then through the mesiobuccal marginal gingiva (▶ Fig. 8.17).

When passing the needle through tissue, the needle should enter the surface of the mucosa at a right angle to make the smallest possible hole in the mucosal flap. If the needle enters soft tissue at an acute angle and is pushed (rather than turned) through tissue, tearing of the mucosa is likely to occur. This will form a crossover, or a figure-8, within the socket (▶ Fig. 8.18).

137

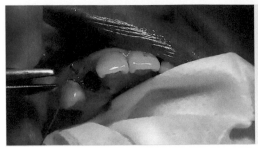

Fig. 8.16 The first pass of the needle when suturing is made faciolingually through the distobuccal marginal gingiva toward its mesiopalatal counterpart.

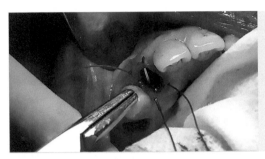

Fig. 8.17 The needle is then passed through the distopalatal marginal gingiva then through the mesiobuccal marginal gingiva.

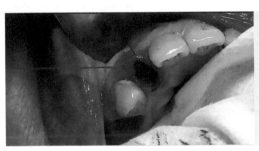

Fig. 8.18 The formation of a crossover suture, or a figure-8, within the socket.

When passing the needle through the flap, the surgeon must ensure that an adequate amount of tissue is taken to prevent the needle or suture from pulling through the soft tissue flap. Because the flap being sutured is a mucoperiosteal flap, it should not be tied too tightly. The minimal amount of tissue between the suture and the edge of the flap should be 3 mm. Presence of significant inflammation in the soft tissues may require a "larger bite" of tissue. Once the sutures are passed through the buccal and lingual tissues, they are tied with an instrument tie (▶ Fig. 8.19 and ▶ Fig. 8.20).

Once the suture knot is tied, it remains on the facial surface of the socket. Note that the size of the opening of the socket is decreased by about 40% (▶ Fig. 8.21).

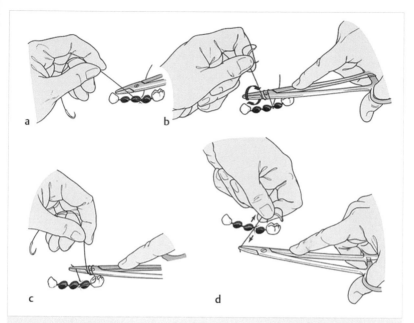

Fig. 8.19 To perform an instrument tie: (**a**) The suture is pulled through tissue until the short tail of the suture (1–2 cm long) remains. The needle holder is held horizontally by the right hand in preparation for the knot-tying procedure. (**b**) The left hand then wraps the long end of the suture around the needle holder twice in the clockwise direction to make two loops of suture around the needle holder. (**c**) The surgeon then opens the needle holder and grasps the short end of the suture very near its end. (**d**) The ends of the suture are then pulled to tighten the knot. The needle holder should not pull the suture it is holding at all until the knot is nearly tied to avoid lengthening that portion of the suture. (From Hupp JR. Principles of More Complex Exodontia. In Hupp JR, Ellis E 3rd, Tucker MR, eds. Contemporary Oral and Maxillofacial Surgery. 6th ed. St. Louis, MO: Mosby Elsevier; 2014:126–127.)

The clot is secured and the patient will be discharged with little to no bleeding. The marginal gingiva is better approximated for rapid epithelialization and closure of the socket.

Place a folded 4″ × 4″ piece of gauze over the extraction site and have the patient bite down gently. This firm pressure will facilitate the formation of a stable blood clot. Ensure hemostasis (no active bleeding) is present before dismissing the patient. Make sure to give the patient postop instructions, an analgesic prescription if necessary, and a follow-up appointment, if necessary.

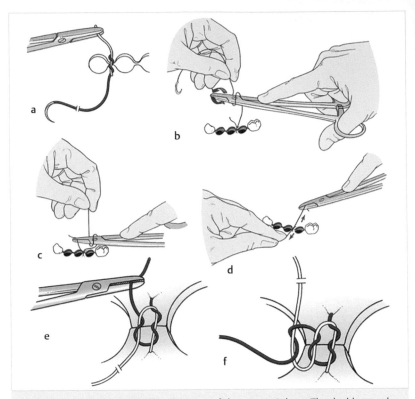

Fig. 8.20 (a) This is the end of the first step of the surgeon's knot. The double wrap has resulted in a double overhand knot. This increases the friction in the knot and will keep the wound edges together until the second portion of the knot is tied. **(b)** The needle holder is then released from the short end of the suture and held in the same position as when the knot-tying procedure began. The left hand then makes a single wrap in the counterclockwise direction. **(c)** The needle holder then grasps the short end of the suture at its end. **(d)** This portion of the knot is completed by pulling this loop firmly down against the previous portion of the knot. **(e)** This completes the surgeon's knot. The double loop of the first pass holds tissue together until the second portion of the square knot can be tied. **(f)** Most surgeons add a third throw to their instrument tie when using a resorbable suture material. The needle holder is repositioned in the original position, and one wrap is placed around the needle holder in the original clockwise direction. The short end of the suture is grasped and tightened down firmly to form the second square knot. The final throw of three knots is tightened firmly. (Note: For demonstration purposes, the first knot is left loose here, but in actual knot tying, the first knot is tightened before creating the second knot.) Both ends of the suture are now cut, leaving about 1 cm or less of the suture end with the knot. (From Hupp JR. Principles of More Complex Exodontia. In Hupp JR, Ellis E 3rd, Tucker MR, eds. Contemporary Oral and Maxillofacial Surgery. 6th ed. St. Louis, MO: Mosby Elsevier; 2014:126–127.)

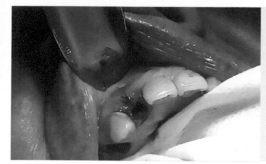

Fig. 8.21 Once the suture knot is tied, it remains on the facial surface of the socket. Note that the size of the opening of the socket is decreased by about 40%.

Extraction Procedure—Surgical Extraction

Indications for Surgical Extractions

- Perform a surgical extraction in the following cases:
  - Severe loss of crown structure.
  - A rigid tooth that cannot be luxated with extraction forceps.
  - Widely divergent roots—tooth will not elevate without risking fracture or loss of bone.
  - Dense, unyielding surrounding bone (such as lateral exostoses).
  - Nearby structures that must be visualized and protected (such as severely crowded teeth).
  - Unplanned crown fracture during a simple extraction procedure.

Surgical Extraction Technique

Develop a Soft-Tissue Flap

Using a #15 blade, make a sulcular incision parallel to the long axis of the tooth to be removed. The incision should be made on the facial surface of the tooth. The blade is inserted into the gingival sulcus and is pressed down to the level of the bone. This creates an incision through gingival epithelium, gingival connective tissue, and periosteum. The incision should extend both at least one tooth anterior and posterior to the tooth to be removed.

Principles of Soft-Tissue Flap Design

- The base (apical end) of the flap must be wider than the coronal end of the flap.
  - This preserves the blood supply to the coronal end of the flap.
  - Blood supply in the gingiva is more linear and vertical in nature.

- Keratinized mucosa heals more rapidly and comfortably than nonkeratinized mucosa.
- Vertical releasing incisions should be placed at least one tooth anterior or posterior to the site of interest.
  - This allows suturing of the flap to take place over intact bone rather than over an empty socket.
  - This prevents the soft tissue from collapsing and dehiscing (opening) during the healing phase.
  - Make vertical releasing incisions parallel to the local vasculature.
    - Include a papilla at the apex of the flap, perpendicular to the gingival margin at line angles of teeth.
  - In many cases, simply making the initial incision longer (spanning more teeth) will eliminate the need for vertical releasing incisions.
    - This can be helpful, as vertical releasing incisions cause more patient pain and discomfort, and are significantly more difficult to suture.
    - Changes in papilla anatomy can be problematic in the esthetic zone as well.
- Remove bone conservatively around the tooth, if necessary.
  - This allows elevator access to the periodontal ligament space.
  - Make troughs with a bur around the crestal margin of the tooth.
    - A #702 or #703 bur in an electric surgical hand piece is commonly used.
  - Avoid the periodontal ligament or tooth structure of the adjacent teeth.
  - As a last resort, or if part of a necessary alveoloplasty, remove part of the facial plate of bone.
- Section the tooth with a hand piece.
  - A #702 or #703 bur is commonly used.
  - Stop short of completely sectioning through the tooth to avoid perforating the lingual cortical plate.
    - Complete the section of the final 1–2 mm via forced separation with an elevator (#77 R elevator works well).
  - Sectioning patterns:
    - Upper first and second molars—use a "Y" pattern: with the stem passing between the two buccal roots and the branches passing toward the mesiopalatal and distopalatal around the palatal root.
    - Lower molars—buccolingual: between the mesial and distal roots.
    - Upper bicuspids—mesiodistal and deep to enter the furcation near the apex and be mindful of the adjacent teeth.
    - Other conical-rooted teeth—mesiodistally or buccolingually and deep.
- Complete the sectioning of the tooth with a straight (#301 or bayonet) or angled (#77 R) elevator inserted into the slot created by the surgical bur in the tooth structure.

- Elevate the tooth fragments with a succession of elevators starting with either a bayonet elevator or a small straight elevator (#301), and then a larger, angled elevator (#77 R).
- A Blumenthal rongeur can be very useful for individual root removal.
- Examine the root pieces for complete removal.
- Inspect the socket for remaining pieces of tooth or exposure of the sinus, inferior alveolar nerve, or perforations of the cortical plates.
- Using copious amounts of saline, irrigate within the socket and under the mucoperiosteal soft-tissue flap to remove gross bone and tooth debris.
- Ensure hemostasis; if needed, consider the use of Gelfoam®, bone burnishing, firm pressure, and sutures.
  - Use Gelfoam® or a similar procoagulant resorbable product for all patients on anticoagulants, including 81 mg aspirin (see Chapter 11, Management of Patients on Anticoagulant and Antiplatelet Medications).
- Suturing (▶ Table 8.1):
  - 3–0 chromic is preferred; but if using a nonresorbable suture material (nylon or silk), plan to remove sutures 7 to 10 days after surgery.

Postoperative Instructions

- Bite on a folded 4″ × 4″ gauze for 20 minutes.
- Urge caution to prevent biting the cheek, lip, or tongue while still anesthetized.
- Advise against aggressive mouth rinsing on the day of surgery to avoid dislodging the blood clot.
- Red-colored saliva may be apparent for 12 to 24 hours and is normal.
- If necessary, prescribe or recommend nonsteroidal anti-inflammatory medications.
- Drinking fluids (but not aggressively rinsing) is encouraged (avoid hot liquids on the first day).
- Encourage a soft diet (e.g., soups, Jell-O, scrambled eggs, pancakes, mashed potatoes).
- Slight swelling may be expected after removal of teeth.
  - It is normal for facial swelling to reach its peak 48 to 72 hours after surgery.
- Sinus precautions (only if an oral-antral communication occurred):
  - Do not blow the nose on the affected side for 7 to 10 days.
  - Sneeze through the mouth instead of the nose for 7 to 10 days.
  - No smoking or sucking through straws for 7 to 10 days.
  - Avoid playing wind instruments for 7 to 10 days.
- Call the office/clinic if questions or concerns arise.

Table 8.1 Suture material

Suture	Type	Raw material	Tensile strength	Absorption rate	Tissue reaction	Contraindications	Frequent uses
Gut	Plain and chromic	Collagen derived from healthy cattle and sheep	Individual patient characteristics can affect rate of tensile strength	Absorbed by proteolytic enzymatic digestive process	Moderate	Should not be used where extended approximation of tissues under stress is required; do not use in patients with known allergy to collagen or chromium	Soft tissue closure
Silk	Braided	Organic protein called fibroin	Progressive degradation of fiber may result in gradual loss of tensile strength over time	Gradual encapsulation by fibrous connective tissue	Acute inflammatory reaction	Do not use in patients with known allergy to silk	Soft tissue closure
Nylon	Monofilament	Long-chain aliphatic polymers	Progressive hydrolysis may result in a gradual loss of tensile strength over time	Gradual encapsulation by fibrous connective tissue	Minimal inflammatory reaction	Should not be used where permanent retention of tensile strength is required	Soft tissue closure

Postoperative Indications for Antibiotics

- Increased risk for local infection (consider prophylactic antibiotics in lieu of postop):
  - Immunocompromised.
  - Immunosuppressed.
- Evidence of preoperative local infection:
  - Swelling/cellulitis.
  - Erythema (redness).
  - Fever.
  - Lymphadenopathy.
  - Purulence in the surgical site.
  - Pericoronitis.
- Prolonged surgery or improper aseptic technique (antibiotics should be considered).

Healing Process Following Extraction

Extraction Socket—Normal Healing Process Timeline

Time period	Expected healing
First few hours	Stable blood clot fills socket; hemostasis achieved.
48 hours	Infiltration of clot with organizing soft tissue and collagen deposition.
4 days	Decreased fibrin content of clot; organizing soft tissue; marginal epithelium migrates apically.
1 week	Diffuse islands of osteoid lined by osteoblasts fill the tissue. Epithelial healing from the gingival peripheral over the clot.
2 weeks	Spicules of bone lined by osteoblasts without osteocytes. Healing of soft tissue over clot complete.
4 weeks	Larger spicules of lamellar bone come together. Depression of gingiva over the healing extraction socket.
8 weeks	Larger blocks of compact bone with area of osteoid around the forming bone ringed by osteoblasts.
12 weeks	Amount of cancellous bone increasing with active remodeling. Complete fill of extraction socket with bone.
16 weeks	Cancellous bone in socket continuously remodeling.

Impaired Healing

- Causes: "4 Ms"
  - Malignancy.
  - Metabolic deficiency.
  - Manipulation.
  - Mobility.
- Glucocorticoids delay healing by interfering with migration of polymorphonuclear leukocytes and macrophages.
- Poor vascularity in area around the wound, anemia, dehydration, increased age, infection, and diabetes mellitus can all slow the healing process.

Complications of Dentoalveolar Procedures

Alveolar Osteitis (Dry Socket)

- Develops on the 2nd to 5th postoperative day.
- Etiology:
  - Increased fibrinolytic activity.
  - Loss of blood clot.
  - Not an infectious process and should not be treated with antibiotics.
- Risk factors for dry socket:
  - Patient age > 25 years.
  - Smoking.
  - Oral contraceptive use.
  - Experience of surgeon.
  - Female patient.
- Signs of dry socket:
  - Worsening, throbbing pain.
  - Radiation of pain to ear and/or chin on affected side.
  - Fetid odor.
  - Bad taste.
  - Poorly-healed extraction site.
- The goal of treatment is to manage the patient's pain during the healing phase.
- Treatment of dry socket (may need to administer local anesthesia in order to comfortably treat):
  - Irrigation of the affected socket with normal saline or sterile water.
  - Placement of sedative dressing (eugenol-based) into the affected socket.
  - The sedative dressing is to be changed every 24 to 48 hours until the patient is asymptomatic (typically 3–4 days).
  - It is important to avoid multiple repeated packings of the socket with foreign materials, as this may lead to complications such as foreign body reactions or chronic bone infections.

- Alveolar osteitis, while painful, will heal given time even without any treatment other than pain management.
- Control pain (analgesic drugs):
  o Nonsteroidal anti-inflammatory medications (*preferred*). Example, ibuprofen 400 to 600 mg every 6 to 8 hours as needed for pain; typically for 1 to 3 days.
  o Narcotic combination analgesic medications. Example, Tylenol #3 (300 mg acetaminophen and 30 mg codeine): 1 tab by mouth (PO) every 6 to 8 hours (q6–8h) as needed for (prn) pain; typically for 1 to 3 days.
- Curettage or over-manipulation of the site not recommended.

Root Fracture/Fragments and Root Tips

- If retrieval attempts are unsuccessful, three conditions must exist for a tooth fragment/root tip to be left in place:
  - The retained root should not be greater than 5 mm in length.
  - The retained root must be embedded in bone.
  - The tooth involved must not be infected (no caries/periapical infection/ pathology).

Root Displacement
Maxillary Sinus

- Most often the palatal root of the maxillary first molar is the culprit.
- If the fragment is 3 mm or less without pre-existing sinus disease, minimal attempts to remove the displaced root should be attempted.
- Local measures are as follows:
  - Have the patient gently blow his/her nose with the nostrils held closed.
  - Utilize fine tip suction with good lighting in an attempt to retrieve tooth root.
  - Antral lavage with suction—irrigate saline through the socket to fill the sinus.
  - Pack iodoform gauze in antrum in attempt to grab the root in gauze.
- If local measures fail, Caldwell-Luc surgical approach affords good visualization.
  - Typically, these procedures are best performed by oral and maxillofacial surgeons (OMSs); therefore, a referral should be considered.
- Sinus precautions, antibiotics, nasal spray decongestant (e.g., oxymetazoline HCl) should be prescribed to prevent infection and to keep the ostium open.

Submandibular Space

- Lingual cortical bone becomes thinner posteriorly in the mandible.
- Attempt to place pressure on the lingual plate to tease the root fragment through the fractured socket site with the aid of a root tip pick.

- If conservative therapy fails, a lingual flap with careful dissection can be attempted.
- Consider abandonment of retrieval if the surgical attempt is extensive and endangers surrounding structures/nerves.

Oral Antral Communications

- 2 mm or less: the patient should be placed on sinus precautions.
  - No nose blowing for 7 to 10 days.
  - Sneeze through the mouth for 7 to 10 days.
  - Avoid using straws for 7 to 10 days.
  - Avoid smoking for 7 to 10 days.
  - Avoid wind instruments for 7 to 10 days.
  - Antibiotics for 7 to 10 days.
    - Consider amoxicillin/clavulanic acid if not penicillin allergic. Augmentin® 500 mg: 1 tab by mouth 3 times daily for 7 to 10 days.
  - Nasal decongestant.
    - e.g., oxymetazoline HCl. Afrin® nasal spray: 2 puffs per naris twice daily for 72 hours.
- 3 to 4 mm: closely approximate gingival tissues, placement of oxidized cellulose as a patch over the communication, and place figure-8 suture to encourage blood clot.
- 5 mm or greater: consider flap procedure for closure.
  - If not comfortable performing such a procedure, consider referral to an OMS.
- Sequelae of oroantral communication:
  - Chronic oroantral fistula.
  - Maxillary sinusitis/pansinusitis.
- Nasal decongestants and antibiotics are recommended for oroantral communications greater than 2 mm.

Tuberosity Fracture

- The maxillary tuberosity is important for maxillary denture reconstruction and retention.
- If the tuberosity fractures while removing a tooth, but remains attached to overlying periosteum, use finger support to retain the tuberosity segment while tooth is extracted.
- If the tuberosity is excessively mobile, stabilize the tooth with a splint and defer extraction for 6 to 8 weeks to allow for tuberosity healing.
- The tooth should (then) be removed surgically by raising a flap, removing a small, but necessary, amount of buccal bone and dividing the tooth into separate roots.

- If the tuberosity is completely separated from the overlying soft tissues, remove it and smooth the surrounding bone with a bone file prior to placement of sutures.

Bleeding

- If the patient is at high risk for bleeding, establish a medical consult prior to ceasing anticoagulant medication.
- Aspirin (ASA) or antiplatelet medications may be held only if tolerated by the patient's medical condition and *ordered by their medical doctor* (MD).
- Warfarin use: consult the patient's MD to reduce international normalized ratio (INR) level to a safe operative level (INR < 3.5–4.0 is usually sufficient as long as local measures are taken to ensure hemostasis).
- Importantly, there is no evidence that antiplatelet therapy increases oral surgical or other surgical bleeding risk.
- In most instances, it is prudent to continue antiplatelet therapy.
- Heparin: defer surgery until 6 hours after heparin has been stopped.
- Pressure hemostasis should be attempted on all patients for up to 30 minutes.
- Local mechanical hemostatic agents.
  - Absorbable gelatin sponge (e.g., Gelfoam®).
    - Secure in socket with figure-8 suture.
    - Scaffold for blood blot formation.
  - Oxidized regenerated cellulose (e.g., Surgicel®).
    - Provides scaffold.
    - Bactericidal in vitro against a wide range of gram-positive and gram-negative organisms.
    - Associated neurotoxicity in intra-alveolar nerve exposure.
    - Associated with delayed wound healing.
  - Collagen: promotes platelet aggregation.
    - Microfibrillar collagen (e.g., Avitene®).
    - Collaplug—highly cross-linked collagen.
  - Tannin: aids in blood clot formation.
    - Chemical trigger for blood clot formation.
    - Present in black tea bags, which may be utilized at home.
    - Used for secondary bleeds.
    - Hold for 30 minutes.
  - Chitosan-derived bandage: (e.g., HemCon®).
    - Positively charged chitosan attracts red blood cells which have negative charges.
    - The red blood cells create a seal over the wound as they are drawn into the bandage, forming a seal and activating additional coagulation pathways.

149

Periodontal Defect

- Risk of decreased socket bone fill increases with age.
- Patients < 25 years of age are at virtually no risk.
  - Predictably fill extraction sockets with bone.
- Patients > 25 years of age are at 30% risk of increased pocket depth.
  - Insufficient socket bone fill.
- Twenty-five percent of patients with retained asymptomatic third molars have considerable periodontal disease in the region.

Nerve Dysfunction and Injuries

- There are reported risk rates to the various branches of the mandibular nerve after performing different types of oral surgical procedures.
  - 0.4 to 11.5% *temporary* sensory deficits.
  - 0.1 to 1% *permanent* sensory deficits.
- Increased lingual nerve paresthesia associated with raising of a lingual flap in the posterior molar region.
- Experience of the operator can contribute to lingual and inferior alveolar nerve paresthesia.
- Inferior alveolar nerve injury is more associated with the following panoramic radiographic findings:
  - Diversion of the inferior alveolar canal.
  - Darkening and narrowing of the third molar root.
  - Interruption of the cortical lines of the inferior alveolar canal.
- Third molar angulation (mesioangular, distoangular, vertical) is not associated with increased risk to the nerve.
- Types of nerve dysfunction include:
  - Anesthesia: Complete loss of sensation.
  - Paresthesia/hypoesthesia: Partial loss of sensation (tingling, tickling).
  - Hyperesthesia: Increased perception of a normal stimulus.
  - Dysesthesia: Painful sensation to normal stimulus (burning, zinging, lancinating).
  - Neurapraxia:
    - Mild injury with no axonal damage.
    - Spontaneous recovery within 4 weeks.
  - Axonotmesis:
    - Axonal damage but intact endoneural and perineural sheath.
    - Wallerian degeneration distal to injury.
    - Potential for recovery in 1 to 3 months.
  - Neurotmesis:
    - Complete severance of axon with gap.
    - No recovery expected without surgery.
    - Recovery can occur if the ends of the nerve are in close approximation (e.g., inferior alveolar canal).

Other Complications of Dentoalveolar Surgery

- Pain.
- Infection/cellulitis.
- Edema (swelling).
- Aspiration of tooth or foreign objects.
- Mucosa laceration.
- Air (cervicofacial) emphysema, often caused by air from nonsurgical, air-driven dental handpieces.
  – Regular dental handpieces are contraindicated for tooth removal.
- Temporomandibular discomfort/injuries/trismus.
  – The use of an appropriately-sized bite block may minimize risk.
- Jaw fracture (mandible, tuberosity, alveolar bone).
  – The presence of a third molar increases the risk of a mandibular angle fracture 2.8-fold.
- Damage to adjacent teeth.
- Displacement of root fragments or teeth into:
  – Mandibular canal.
  – Infratemporal fossa.
  – Lateral pterygoid space.
- Aggressive hemorrhage from an anomalous vessel.
- Displacement of maxillary third molar into the maxillary sinus or infratemporal fossa.
- Displacement of mandibular third molar lingually into submandibular/lateral pterygoid spaces.

Clinical Pearls

- Acute infection is NOT a contraindication to extraction (but remember local anesthetic and pH principles).
- The palatal root of the maxillary first molar is the most common root to be accidentally displaced into the maxillary sinus.

Third Molars

Classifications for Third Molars

- Winter's classification of impacted third molars is based on the radiographic appearance of the third molar and its anatomical position in relation to the long axis of the second molar.
  – Mesioangular.
  – Distoangular.
  – Vertical.

– Horizontal.
– Buccoangular.
– Linguoangular.
– Inverted.

Third Molars—Indications for Removal

• Pain-free does not necessarily mean problem- or pathology-free when it comes to third molars.
• Third molars (wisdom teeth) are typically the last teeth/molars to grow in the late teen years.
• Even wisdom teeth that are not causing pain (symptom-free) pose an increased risk for chronic oral infections, periodontitis, and tooth decay, according to results of a 7-year clinical trial conducted by researchers for the American Association of Oral and Maxillofacial Surgeons (AAOMS).
• Wisdom teeth require removal when they are unable to properly erupt in the mouth.
• They may grow sideways, emerge only partially, or even remain trapped beneath the gingiva and bone (this is termed "impacted").
• Impacted teeth can cause many health problems including tumors or cysts around the roots that can destroy the jawbone and nearby healthy teeth.
• Partially erupted teeth may allow bacteria to grow, potentially leading to gum disease (gingivitis or periodontitis) that causes swelling, stiffness, pain, and illness.
• Oral bacteria associated with periodontal disease have been linked to more serious health problems, including coronary artery disease, stroke, kidney disease, and diabetes.
• The "Third Molar Clinical Trials" research added a new perspective to the possible risks for young women.
• Periodontitis affecting retained wisdom teeth can lead to inflammation throughout the body, increasing the risk of delivering a low-birth-weight infant.
• Third molars often push adjacent teeth out of alignment, thereby altering the bite and threatening jaw integrity.
• Many orthodontists refer their patients to an OMS for third molar removal before beginning treatment to minimize the risk of gingivitis and other problems that could affect the success of the orthodontia.
• In general, a young adult's wisdom teeth have incomplete root development, making tooth removal relatively uncomplicated.
• As wisdom teeth continue to grow, however, the roots lengthen and may become tangled or intimately in contact with the sensory nerves that run through the mandible (mandibular nerve) or the sinus area.
• While not all wisdom teeth may need to be removed, all of them need to be managed.

- The best advice for management of third molars is dependent on a thorough examination, appropriate imaging, and discussions with the patient and/or responsible family members.
- If a decision is made to retain the wisdom teeth, patients are advised to keep the areas meticulously clean and get an annual examination to assess any changes in the teeth or gingiva.

When are Third Molars Recommended for Removal?

- Patient has symptoms of pain, bleeding, swelling, bad taste, or drainage.
- Patient < 25 years of age with one episode of pericoronitis.
- Patient < 25 years of age with a periodontal defect on the adjacent second molar.
- Patient 26 to 40 years of age with repeated episodes of pericoronitis.
- Patient 26 to 40 years of age with periodontal pockets > 4 mm.
- Patient > 40 years of age with presence of purulence (pus).
- Patient > 40 years of age with presence of pathology.
- AAOMS supports routine intervention on third molars.
  - Evidence of the incidence of problems/pathology associated with impacted third molars is sufficient enough to warrant their removal when they are currently "asymptomatic."

Periodontal Considerations in Third Molar Removal

- The presence of impacted third molars adversely affects the periodontium of adjacent second molars as reflected in disruption of the periodontal ligament, root resorption, and pocket depth associated with loss of attachment.
- Removal of impacted third molars can lead to periodontal defects around adjacent second molars.
  - The preoperative existence of an intrabony defect, age of the patient, and level of plaque control may serve to predict adverse outcomes.
- The presence of visible third molars is associated with overall elevated levels of periodontitis and that of immediately adjacent teeth.
- In the presence of visible third molars, periodontitis involving adjacent teeth is progressive and only partially responsive to therapy.
- The evaluation of a visible third molar for removal should include an assessment of the periodontium associated with both the third molar itself and that of adjacent teeth, and include anatomical limitations to mechanical removal of plaque.
- The presence of pocket depths of ≥ 4 to 5 mm and/or bleeding on probing should be recognized as possible predictors of future progression of periodontitis.

- Support for the hypothesis that third molars should be considered as a possible predictor of periodontitis include:
  - The association of overall increased disease severity in the presence of visible third molars.
  - The progressive nature of periodontitis involving non-third molars when third molars are present.
  - The relationship between visible third molars and bacteria associated with severe and refractory periodontitis.
  - The negative impact of visible third molars on treatment outcomes.

The Microflora around the Second and Third Molars

- Data on microflora and asymptomatic disease in the third molar region show:
  - Absence of symptoms does not indicate absence of disease or pathology.
  - Pathogenic bacteria in clinically significant numbers exist in and around asymptomatic third molars.
  - Periodontal disease as indicated by probing depths > 4 mm exists in and around asymptomatic third molars.
  - Indicators of chronic inflammation exist in periodontal pockets in and around asymptomatic third molars.
  - Periodontal disease progresses in the absence of symptoms.

The Effects of Age on Various Parameters Relating to Third Molars

- Periodontal defects, as assessed by pocket depths, deteriorate with increasing age in the presence of retained third molars.
- Caries in erupted third molars increase in prevalence with increasing age.
- The incidence of postoperative morbidity following third molar removal is higher in patients > 25 years of age.
- Germectomy may be associated with a lower incidence of postoperative morbidity.

Role of Coronectomy in Third Molar Removal

- Coronectomy refers to partial odontectomy and removal of the impacted tooth's crown only, with the nonenamel structures remaining in the socket.
- When imaging suggests an intimate relationship between the roots of the mandibular third molar and the inferior alveolar nerve and the tooth still needs to be treated, consideration should be given to coronectomy with retention of the portion of the roots associated with the inferior alveolar nerve.

- Contraindications:
  - Periapical infection.
  - Mobile roots.
  - Caries that extends to the pulp.
  - Angulation of tooth that would place the inferior alveolar nerve/lingual nerve at risk; for example, horizontal or lingual version over lingual plate.

Bibliography

[1] AAOMSRO. OMS Reference Guide. 3rd ed. Rosemont, IL: AAOMS; 2013

[2] AAOMS White Paper on Third Molar Data. Rosemont, IL: American Association of Oral and Maxillofacial Surgeons; 2007. Available at: http://www.aaoms.org/docs/govt_affairs/advocacy_white_papers/white_paper_third_molar_data.pdf. Accessed Feb 25, 2017

[3] Andreasen JO, Bakland LK, Flores MT, et al. Traumatic Dental Injuries: A Manual. 3rd ed. Ames, IA: Wiley Blackwell; 2011

[4] Bataineh AB. Sensory nerve impairment following mandibular third molar surgery. J Oral Maxillofac Surg. 2001; 59(9):1012–1017, discussion 1017

[5] Blaeser BF, August MA, Donoff RB, Kaban LB, Dodson TB. Panoramic radiographic risk factors for inferior alveolar nerve injury after third molar extraction. J Oral Maxillofac Surg. 2003; 61 (4):417–421

[6] Blakey GH, Marciani RD, Haug RH, et al. Periodontal pathology associated with asymptomatic third molars. J Oral Maxillofac Surg. 2002; 60(11):1227–1233

[7] Carter G, Goss AN, Lloyd J, Tocchetti R. Current concepts of the management of dental extractions for patients taking warfarin. Aust Dent J. 2003; 48(2):89–96, quiz 138

[8] Curran AE, Damm DD, Drummond JF. Pathologically significant pericoronal lesions in adults: Histopathologic evaluation. J Oral Maxillofac Surg. 2002; 60(6):613–617, discussion 618

[9] Dodson TB. Is there a role for reconstructive techniques to prevent periodontal defects after third molar surgery? J Oral Maxillofac Surg. 2005; 63(7):891–896

[10] Elo JA, Sun HH, Dong F, Tandon R, Singh HM. Novel incision design and primary flap closure reduces the incidence of alveolar osteitis and infection in impacted mandibular third molar surgery. Oral Surg Oral Med Oral Pathol Oral Radiol. 2016; 122(2):124–133

[11] Elo JA, Sun HB, Dong F, Nguyen K, Zakhary K. Does bone grafting improve outcomes in coronectomy surgery? Long-term (5- to 9-year) clinical and radiographic follow-up of 78 adult patients. J Oral Maxillofac Surg. 2017; 75(7):1330–1337

[12] Eshghpour M, Nezadi A, Moradi A, Shamsabadi RM, Rezaei NM, Nejat A. Pattern of mandibular third molar impaction: A cross-sectional study in northeast of Iran. Niger J Clin Pract. 2014; 17(6):673–677

[13] Halmos DR, Ellis E, III, Dodson TB. Mandibular third molars and angle fractures. J Oral Maxillofac Surg. 2004; 62(9):1076–1081

[14] Hupp JR. Principles of management of impacted teeth. In: Hupp JR, Ellis E 3rd, Tucker MR, eds. Contemporary Oral and Maxillofacial Surgery. 5th ed. St. Louis, MO: Mosby Elsevier; 2008: 153–178

[15] Hupp JR. Principles of more complex exodontia. In: Hupp JR, Ellis E 3rd, Tucker MR, eds. Contemporary Oral and Maxillofacial Surgery. 6th ed. St. Louis, MO: Mosby Elsevier; 2014: 126–127

[16] Nance PE, White RP, Jr, Offenbacher S, Phillips C, Blakey GH, Haug RH. Change in third molar angulation and position in young adults and follow-up periodontal pathology. J Oral Maxillofac Surg. 2006; 64(3):424–428

[17] Ventä I, Ylipaavalniemi P, Turtola L. Clinical outcome of third molars in adults followed during 18 years. J Oral Maxillofac Surg. 2004; 62(2):182–185

9 Antibiotics

Rawle F. Philbert, Jeffrey A. Elo, Alan S. Herford, Ho-Hyun Sun, Christopher H. Yi

Antibiotic Types

- Penicillins (e.g., penicillin, amoxicillin)
- Cephalosporins (e.g., cephalexin)
- Macrolides (e.g., erythromycin, clarithromycin, azithromycin)
- Fluoroquinolones (e.g., ciprofloxacin, levofloxacin)
- Sulfonamides (e.g., sulfamethoxazole, trimethoprim)
- Tetracyclines (e.g., tetracycline, doxycycline)
- Aminoglycosides (e.g., gentamicin, tobramycin)

Principles of Antibiotic Dosing

- The objective is to help the body's defenses clear tissues of pathogenic microorganisms by achieving levels in the infected sites that are equal or greater than the minimum inhibitory concentrations (MIC).
- Eliminate the causative agents physically (incision and drainage).
  - Odontogenic infections rarely rebound, particularly if the source of the infection has been eliminated (root canal or extraction).
- The pathogenic organisms must be susceptible to the antimicrobial agent.
- There should be sufficient drug concentration at the site of infection during the course of therapy.
- Local factors that may interfere with the drug's effect must be minimized.
- Antibiotics should be used aggressively and for a sufficient duration of time to result in clinical improvement/resolution.
- Host defenses must be adequate for the eventual eradication of pathogens and associated toxins.

Antibiotic Loading Doses

- Most odontogenic infections begin and peak rapidly.
- High antibiotic level must be reached quickly.
  - This is achieved by loading doses.
  - Loading doses are two to four times the maintenance doses.
  - If a loading dose is not used, approximately four maintenance doses spaced at the recommended intervals are required to achieve a steady-state blood level of the antibiotic.
- For antibiotics with exceptional bioavailability (e.g., amoxicillin), a loading dose is not as crucial as it is with penicillin V or cephalexin, which are not absorbed as readily.

Antibiotic Dosing Variables

- Diffusion to the infection site:
  - Diffusion through capillary endothelium is easy for metronidazole.
  - Diffusion is difficult for beta-lactams and aminoglycosides, while tetracyclines and fluoroquinolones demonstrate intermediate diffusion profiles.
- Lipid solubility:
  - Lipophilic agents (e.g., tetracyclines, macrolides, and fluoroquinolones) pass through barriers (such as cellular membranes) better than hydrophilic beta-lactams and aminoglycosides.
- Plasma protein binding ability:
  - Lower plasma protein binding may be preferred (e.g., amoxicillin vs. penicillin VK) because they pass more readily.
- Inoculum effect:
  - The principle that antibiotics lose efficacy against a dense mass of microbial population.
  - May significantly affect antibiotic activity and the ability of the drug to penetrate to the core of infection.
    - This is the benefit of incision and drainage.
- Surface/volume ratio:
  - Incision and drainage generate a high vascularity, low infection volume situation.
  - This promotes better antibiotic penetration.
- Pregnancy.
  - Most antibiotics commonly used in dentistry are safe for the pregnant patient; but there is potential for some to harm the developing baby.
  - It is not uncommon for patients to require antibiotics to treat a dental infection while pregnant.
  - Some antibiotics are known to be teratogenic and should be avoided entirely during pregnancy.
    - These include streptomycin and kanamycin (may cause hearing loss) and tetracycline (can lead to weakening, hypoplasia, and discoloration of long bones and teeth).
  - Recommend and prescribe antibiotics for pregnant patients only if absolutely indicated.
  - If possible, avoid initiating antibiotic therapy during the first trimester, as this is the period of fetal structural development; and therefore, the highest risk for iatrogenic teratogenicity.
  - Select a safe antibiotic medication.
    - This often means selecting an established antibiotic with a proven track record in pregnancy.
  - Whenever clinically indicated, single-agent antibiotic therapy is preferred over polypharmacy.

157

– Narrow-spectrum antibiotics are preferred over broad-spectrum for the treatment of established odontogenic infection.
– Prescribe the lowest effective dose of antibiotic to treat the infection.
– Discourage the use of over-the-counter drugs that may interfere with the efficacy and/or metabolism of prescription antibiotic medications.
• Renal and hepatic functions.
– Renal dysfunction: as a general rule, the dose interval should be increased for concentration-dependent antibiotics and decreased for time-dependent antibiotics.
– Renal insufficiency: some antibiotics do not require dosage adjustments (e.g., clindamycin, azithromycin).

Duration of Antibiotic Dosing

• Antibiotic prescriptions should be initially aggressive but administered for a minimum amount of a time that is compatible with remission of disease.
– The ideal duration is the shortest time that prevents clinical and microbiological relapse.
• Antibiotic success is best determined by clinical symptom improvement.
• Example: prescribe a reasonable regimen (5–7 days) with an initial loading dose (not needed for amoxicillin) and then re-evaluate shortly into the infection (1 or 2 days) and monitor patient's progress until symptoms improve.
• Prolonged antibiotic duration does not destroy resistant organisms.
• Prolonged treatment is not necessary to prevent rebound oral infections.
• Antibiotic dosage and duration cannot be extrapolated from one infection to another.
• There is no guaranteed way to know how long the infection will last.
– Definite treatment of the infection source is the most effective treatment.
• Dosing guidelines do not take into consideration issues related to microbial virulence, anatomic location of the infection, feasibility of incision and drainage, microbial resistance, and status of host defenses.

Concentration- Versus Time-Dependent Effects

• Concentration-dependent effect:
– Some antibiotics are most effective if very high blood concentrations are achieved periodically.
– Examples include:
  ○ Aminoglycosides.
  ○ Metronidazole.
  ○ Fluoroquinolones.

- Time-dependent effect:
  - Effective if blood levels are maintained above MIC for as long as possible.
  - Examples include beta-lactams and vancomycin.
  - The goal of dosing with cell wall synthesis inhibitors is to maximize the time of exposure and maintain the blood and tissue concentrations above the organisms' MIC for as long as possible.
  - Time-dependent effects are better achieved with longer half-life agents (e.g., amoxicillin) than those with shorter half-lives (e.g., penicillin VK, cephalexin).
- In general, the concentration of the antibiotic in the blood should exceed the MIC by a factor of 2 to 8 times to offset tissue barriers that restrict access to the infected site.

Adverse Outcomes Associated with Antibiotic Use

- Allergic reactions: penicillins, sulfa drugs.
- Antibiotic-induced diarrhea and pseudomembranous colitis: amoxicillin, clindamycin.
- Potential for disturbances of endogenous flora and superinfection.
  - Acquisition and transfer of drug-resistant genes: tetracyclines, vancomycin.
- Antibiotic-associated photosensitivity and phototoxicity: sulfonamides, tetracyclines.
- Antibiotic-induced agranulocytosis: sulfonamides, beta-lactams, aminoglycosides, macrolides.
- Long QT interval syndrome: fluoroquinolones, macrolides, clindamycin.
- Antibiotic-associated mania: clarithromycin, fluoroquinolones.

Inappropriate Antibiotic Use in Dentistry

- Antibiotic therapy initiated after surgery to prevent infection that is unlikely to occur or lacks efficacy for this purpose as demonstrated by clinical trials.
- Failure to use prophylactic antibiotics according to the principles established for such use.
- Use of antibiotics as analgesics in endodontics.
- Overuse in situations in which patients are not at risk for metastatic infections.
- Treatment of chronic periodontitis almost completely amenable to mechanical therapy.
- Long-term administration in the management of periodontitis.
- Antibiotic therapy instead of incision and drainage.
- Antibiotic recommendation for avoiding claims of negligence.
- Administration of antibiotics in improper situations, dosage, and duration of therapy can lead to antibiotic resistance.

159

Antibiotic Resistance

- According to the CDC, at least 2 million Americans are infected each year with bacteria that are resistant to antibiotics.
  - Of these, 23,000 or more die as a result of these infections.
- Inappropriate use of antibiotics is the major culprit.
- Challenge: maintain and preserve the efficacy of current antibiotics.
  - Antibiotic development is not an easy task.
  - All microbial resistance is local (i.e., related to use in a particular community).
  - Antibiotics are societal drugs that cumulatively affect the individual receiving the drug and many others.
- Microbial resistance accelerates when subtherapeutic doses are used.
  - This gives bacteria opportunity to react via mutation, acquisition, or transfer of resistance genes, virulence factors, or expression of latent resistance (also known as induction).
  - The gastrointestinal tract is a massive reservoir for resistance genes readily transferred within and between enteric microbial species, a process greatly enhanced by antibiotics and agents such as tetracyclines, imipenem, cefoxitin, and clavulanic acid.
  - Tissue levels should ideally contain 8- to 10-fold the MIC of an antimicrobial agent to reduce or prevent the emergence of resistant subpopulations.
    - Unfortunately, this is often impossible because of complications or toxic side effects of many antibiotic classes.
- Known evasion mechanisms for antibiotics:
  - Enzymatic inactivation (e.g., beta-lactams, acetyltransferases).
  - Modification or occlusion of the target site (e.g., penicillin-binding proteins for penicillins and DNA gyrase for fluoroquinolones).
  - Ribosomal point mutation (e.g., macrolides, clindamycin).
  - Limitation of antibiotic diffusion often via alteration of cell membrane permeability (e.g., beta-lactams, fluoroquinolones).
  - Active drug efflux (e.g., tet genes effect efflux of tetracyclines out of microbes).
  - Decreased activation of antibiotic compounds (e.g., metronidazole).
  - Overproduction of target sites (e.g., sulfonamides; overproduction of beta-lactamase).

Antibiotic Combinations

- Disadvantages typically outweigh benefits:
  - Greater chance of inducing microbial resistance.
  - Increased likelihood of adverse reactions.
  - Increased costs.
  - Possible pharmacologic antagonism or interference.
  - Greater spread of resistance genes.

- Increased risk of superficial infections (appearance of a new infection when treating a primary one).
- The antagonisms of some combinations are well-documented (e.g., cell wall synthesis inhibitors and protein synthesis inhibitors; protein synthesis inhibitors working on the same ribosomal subunits).
- Examples of effective drug combinations include:
  - Amoxicillin and metronidazole.
  - Ampicillin and gentamicin.
  - Beta-lactams and beta-lactamase inhibitors.
  - Sulfonamides and trimethoprim.

Common Reasons for Antibiotic Failure

- Delayed or incorrect diagnosis.
- Failure to eradicate the source of infection surgically.
- Inappropriate choice of antibiotic.
- Blood antibiotic concentration too low.
- Limited vascularity or blood flow.
- Limited infection site penetration.
- Decreased tissue pH or oxygen tension.
- Impaired/inadequate host defenses.
- Patient failure to take antibiotic as prescribed.
- Slow microbial growth.
- Emergence of antibiotic resistance.
- Antibiotic antagonism/interference.

Terminology

- Bacteriostatic: Inhibits bacterial growth.
- Bactericidal: Kills bacteria.
- Sensitivity: Susceptibility to an antimicrobial agent.
- Resistance: An organism's relative tolerance toward an antimicrobial agent.
- Spectrum: The types of microbes against which the drug remains effective.
- Selective toxicity: The selective action of an agent toward a microbe with minimal disruption of the host's physiologic processes.

General Mechanisms of Antimicrobial Action

- Disruption of microbial nucleic acid structure or their synthesis.
  - Antiviral agents:
    - Anti-herpes simplex virus agents: acyclovir, valacyclovir.
    - Anti-human immunodeficiency virus agents: nucleoside inhibitors, non-nucleoside inhibitors, protease inhibitors, entry inhibitors, integrase inhibitors.

- Metronidazole (bactericidal).
- Fluoroquinolones (bactericidal).
- Disruption of the cell membrane structure or their synthesis.
  - Antifungal agents:
    - Nystatin.
    - Amphotericin B.
    - Azoles: clotrimazole, ketoconazole, fluconazole.
- Disruption of folic acid synthesis:
  - Sulfonamides.
  - Trimethoprim.
- Cell wall synthesis inhibitors:
  - Penicillins (bactericidal).
  - Cephalosporins (bactericidal).
  - Vancomycin (bactericidal).
  - Bacitracin (bactericidal).
- Protein synthesis inhibitors:
  - Macrolides (50S subunit).
  - Clindamycin (50S subunit).
  - Tetracyclines (30S subunit).
  - Aminoglycosides (30S subunit) (bactericidal).
  - Erythromycin.
  - Clarithromycin.
  - Azithromycin.
- Other:
  - Chlorhexidine.

Useful Antibiotics in Dentistry

- Cell wall synthesis inhibitors.
  - Penicillins.
  - Cephalosporins.
- Protein synthesis inhibitors.
  - Clindamycin.
  - Macrolides:
    - Erythromycin.
    - Azithromycin.
    - Clarithromycin.
- Disruption of DNA synthesis.
  - Metronidazole.
- Others.
  - Chlorhexidine.

Penicillins

- Mode of action:
  - Inhibit synthesis of the bacterial cell wall.
  - After attaching to its namesake bacterial enzyme (penicillin-binding proteins), penicillin inhibits the protein's transpeptidation reactions that cross-links the peptide chains attached to the backbone of the peptidoglycan.
  - This leads to inactivation of an inhibitor that limits the activity of autolytic, self-destructive enzymes (e.g., autolysin) within the cell wall.
- Spectrum of coverage:
  - Most gram-positive aerobes and anaerobes.
- Resistant strains:
  - *Staphylococcus aureus.*
  - *Bacteroides fragilis.*
  - *Haemophilus influenzae.*
- Examples:
  - Penicillin VK (oral).
    - Well distributed except to the brain, unless the meninges are inflamed.
    - Elimination via the kidneys.
    - It is well absorbed after oral administration.
  - Amoxicillin (oral).
    - Better pharmacokinetic profile than penicillin VK.
    - Some metabolism in the liver.
    - Excreted predominantly by the kidneys.
    - Crosses the placenta.
    - Enters breast milk.
    - Uses: sinus infections, pneumonia, otitis media, skin infections, urinary tract infections.

Penicillinase-Resistant Penicillins

- Methicillin (injection).
- Nafcillin (injection).
- Dicloxacillin (oral).
- Amoxicillin and clavulanic acid (oral).

Mechanisms of Bacterial Penicillin Resistance

- Production of beta-lactamases (also known as penicillinases) by the bacteria.
  - This reduces the permeability of the outer membrane.
- Production of modified penicillin-binding proteins.

- Methods of defeating penicillin resistance.
  - Use of penicillinase-resistant penicillins such as:
    - Methicillin.
    - Dicloxacillin.
  - Combination of a penicillin with a beta-lactamase inhibitor.
    - Amoxicillin + clavulanic acid.

Adverse Reaction to Penicillin—Allergy

- Allergy to penicillin ranges from 0.7 to 8%.
- Between 0.7 and 4% (average 2%) chance of an allergic reaction during any course of penicillin therapy (types I–IV reactions).
- May occur regardless of the route of administration.
- Ninety percent of all fatal anaphylactic reactions occur within the first 60 minutes of exposure.
- Penicillin anaphylaxis accounts for about 75% of all documented anaphylaxis cases each year (400–800 annual deaths in the United States).
- Treatment is IM epinephrine injection (0.3 mg for adults, 0.15 mg for prepubertal children).

Cephalosporins

- Inhibit bacterial cell wall synthesis.
- Bactericidal.
- Classified into four generations.
  - Subsequent generations of cephalosporins demonstrate:
    - Decreased gram positive coverage.
    - Increased gram negative coverage.
    - Increased resistance to beta-lactamase enzyme.
    - Increased susceptibility to gastric acid degradation.
- First generation (e.g., cephalexin).
  - Absorption: Adequate absorption attained following oral administration.
  - Distribution: Readily binds to plasma proteins and is distributed to most tissues outside of the central nervous system.
  - Excretion: Cleared by renal glomerular filtration.
  - Spectrum:
    - Very effective against gram-positive bacteria.
    - Moderately effective against gram-negative bacteria.
  - Recommendation:
    - Although considered an alternate to penicillin, first-generation cephalosporins do not provide an advantage over the use of penicillins for orofacial infections.
  - Great caution should be exercised when considering a cephalosporin for a penicillin-allergic patient.

  – Examples of first generation cephalosporins:
    ○ Cephalexin (oral).
    ○ Cefazolin (parenteral).
- Second generation (cefaclor).
  – Effective against gram-positive bacteria.
  – Good for *B. fragilis*.
  – More effective against gram-negative bacteria than first-generation cephalosporins.

Protein Synthesis Inhibitors

- Bind to either the 50S or the 30S subunit, thus inhibiting translocation.
- Clindamycin.
  – Description:
    ○ A bacteriostatic agent active against most anaerobic bacteria.
    ○ Considered the drug of choice against infections caused by anaerobic bacteria resistant to penicillins.
  – Absorption:
    ○ Almost complete absorption attained after oral administration.
  – Distribution:
    ○ Passes readily into most tissues including bone.
    ○ Actively transported to the intracellular regions of macrophages and polymorphonuclear neutrophils (PMNs) which leads to accumulation in abscesses.
    ○ Crosses the placenta but does not pass through the meninges.
  – Excretion:
    ○ Metabolized in the liver and excreted in bile.
    ○ Dosage should be decreased if the patient is at risk of impaired hepatic function.
  – Adverse effects:
    ○ The most frequent adverse reaction is diarrhea that occurs in 10 to 20% of individuals—This is probably a consequence of direct action of this drug on the intestinal mucosa and microbiota.
    ○ The most important GI complication is pseudomembranous colitis (antibiotic-associated colitis) induced by *Clostridium difficile* (*C. Diff*). This organism is more resistant to clindamycin and survives antibiotic therapy. *C. Diff* colonizes the colon to cause inflammation, pain, and explosive diarrhea that could put a patient at risk for severe dehydration. Recent studies suggest that risk of colitis is poorly founded in immunocompetent individuals.
    ○ Another frequent side effect is the appearance of morbilliform eruption (3 to 5% of individuals).

- Macrolides.
  - One of the safer antibiotics in use.
  - The prototype drug is erythromycin.
  - It is not the drug of choice for typical, primarily anaerobic dental infections, but it is a satisfactory alternative to penicillin in dentistry, particularly in patients allergic to penicillin.
  - Erythromycin is available for oral administration in four forms, but erythromycin ethylsuccinate and erythromycin stearate are more frequently used.
  - Absorption:
    - Erythromycin base is destroyed by gastric acid, so it should be administered in an enteric-coated tablet that is resistant to acids or capsules containing enteric-coated pellets.
    - Erythromycin stearate is less sensitive to gastric acid.
  - Distribution:
    - Spreads to most body tissues, with peak blood level 1 to 4 hours after ingestion.
    - The serum concentrations obtained with the base or with stearate are similar. Estolate concentrations are typically three to four times higher.
  - Excretion:
    - Via urine and bile.
  - Adverse effects:
    - Gastrointestinal symptoms: vomiting, nausea, diarrhea.
- Azithromycin.
  - Broader coverage including gram-positive and gram-negative aerobes, as well as strict anaerobes, such as *Actinobacillus actinomycetemcomitans* and *Porphyromonas gingivalis.*
  - Indications:
    - Mild-to-moderate infections of the upper and lower respiratory tract.
    - Uncomplicated skin infections.
  - Dosage/route/formulations:
    - 5 to 12 mg/kg/day.
    - Tablet: 250, 500, 600 mg.
    - Adult dose: 500 mg bid.
  - Better oral absorption than erythromycin and penetrates tissues well.
  - Concentration is much higher in tissue than in plasma.
    - Very high levels in saliva, bone, and gingiva.
  - Dental consideration:
    - Alternate drug of choice for mild infection due to susceptible organisms in penicillin-allergic patient.
  - May be more active against streptococcal and staphylococcal organisms than erythromycin.
  - Decreased propensity for drug interactions.

- The Food and Drug Administration required changes in labeling to warn about risk of QT prolongation and cardiac arrhythmias.
  - A significantly higher incidence than those taking amoxicillin or those who took no antibiotic.
- Other macrolides and fluoroquinolones can also prolong QT interval.
  - The risk with levofloxacin was not significantly higher than with azithromycin.
- Tetracyclines.
  - Not a first line class of drugs for dentistry.
  - Inhibit collagenase.
  - Doxycycline and minocycline are the best absorbed tetracyclines and can be dosed once or twice a day, which may enhance patient compliance.
  - Tetracyclines chelate calcium ions and stain the dentition.
    - Concurrent intake with calcium-containing compounds (such as milk) may reduce absorption and decrease serum concentration.
  - Uses:
    - May be used for acne prevention, periodontitis—refractory and juvenile—as well as acute necrotizing ulcerative gingivitis.

Disruption of DNA Synthesis

- Metronidazole.
  - Supplement to penicillin in cases of severe or protracted infection.
  - A non-naturally occurring compound derived from nitroimidazole.
  - Effective against obligate anaerobes.
  - Well absorbed orally.
  - Passes readily into most tissues and into saliva.
  - Excretion via renal system.
  - Mode of action:
    - Reduction of nitro group which in turn disrupts DNA synthesis, leading to cell death.
  - Drug combination:
    - Can be combined with a penicillin drug to elicit additive/synergistic effects against susceptible microorganisms.
  - Adverse effects:
    - Toxic reactions with disulfiram.
    - May propagate the effects of ethanol sensitizing agents such as disulfiram that induces hangover-like course of symptoms upon alcohol consumption.
    - Potentiates the effects of anticoagulants.
    - Metallic taste.
    - Nausea.
    - Large doses may cause peripheral neuropathy.

- Recommendation:
  - Should be considered for the penicillin-allergic patient for serious anaerobic infections. It is active against practically all gram-negative anaerobic rods and clostridia and has been used for infections of dental or periodontal origin in individuals allergic to penicillin. In some specific instances, such as acute necrotizing ulcerative gingivitis or very advanced or refractory periodontitis, its use can be considered if antimicrobial susceptibility testing indicates susceptible strains are present.
  - Aerobic and microaerophilic bacteria are usually resistant.

Topical Agents

- Chlorhexidine.
  - Topical antibiotic produced as a liquid solution that can be used pre- or postsurgery.
  - Bisbiguanide cationic molecule which binds strongly to hydroxyapatite of enamel, the organic pellicle on the tooth surface, the alveolar and gingival mucosa, salivary proteins, and bacteria.
    - Slowly converted to its active form.
    - Reduces plaque accumulation, enhances gingival health, and improves healing.
  - Mechanism of action:
    - Microbial inhibitory effects via binding to lipopolysaccharides, thereby affecting membrane transport systems.
    - Inhibition of sugar uptake into bacterial cells.
  - Spectrum of antibacterial activity is broad and nonspecific.
  - Clinical uses:
    - Disinfection of the oral cavity before dental treatment.
    - As an adjunct drug in initial therapy for: (1) rapidly progressive periodontitis, (2) localized juvenile periodontitis.
    - Following periodontal and implant surgery.
    - In handicapped patients with difficulty maintaining hygiene.
  - Adverse effects and toxicity:
    - Development of yellow-brown extrinsic stain of teeth and soft tissues.
    - Desquamative soft-tissue lesions.
    - Impaired taste sensation (mostly for salt).

Signs of infection typically observed prior to initiating antibiotic therapy

- Swelling.
- Redness.
- Pain.
- Warmth.
- Loss of function.
- Elevated temperature.
- Malaise.

Tests/laboratory studies to consider obtaining when treating odontogenic infection and considering antibiotic therapy

- White blood cell count with differential (*is a blood test*).
- Gram stain (*if there is pus present*).
- Culture and sensitivity (*if there is pus present*).
- Blood culture.
- Tissue culture.

Bibliography

[1] Golan DE, Armstrong EJ, Armstrong AW. Principles of Pharmacology: The Pathophysiologic Basis of Drug Therapy. 4th ed. Philadelphia, PA: Wolters Kluwer Health/Lippincott Williams & Wilkins; 2017

[2] Norwitz ER, Greenberg JA. Antibiotics in pregnancy: Are they safe? Rev Obstet Gynecol. 2009; 2(3):135-136

10 Pharmacology for the Dental Practitioner

Steven L. Fletcher, Jeffrey A. Elo, Alan S. Herford, Ho-Hyun Sun, Christopher H. Yi

Introduction

- Anesthesia and sedation in dentistry can have several forms, including:
  - Local anesthesia alone.
  - Oral and/or intranasal sedation.
  - Intramuscular (IM) sedation.
  - Inhalation sedation (nitrous oxide).
  - Intravenous (IV) mild/moderate sedation.
  - IV deep sedation (*used by oral and maxillofacial surgeons [OMSs]*).
  - Total IV general anesthesia (*used by OMSs*).
  - Inhalation general anesthesia with/without endotracheal intubation.
- Each of these modalities requires complex training and performance by qualified practitioners, as well as a thorough understanding of pharmacology.

This chapter only discusses local anesthesia, nitrous oxide, and medications used for mild/moderate sedation.

Pharmacology

- The field of medical science which deals with the properties and effects of drugs as well as their interactions with living systems such as cells, organs, animals, and humans.

Drug Distribution

- Eventual placement of the drug within the body over a given period of time.
- Primary compartments include:
  - Brain.
  - Muscle.
  - Fat.

Metabolism

- Alteration of the drug by the body.
- Most drugs are metabolized in the liver.
  - Microsomal enzyme alteration (cytochrome [CYP] P-450).
  - Many drugs can inhibit the CYP isoforms of the P-450 drug metabolism system.

- Two simultaneous doses of drugs normally metabolized in this manner may cause elevated blood levels of one or both medications, leading to toxic overdose effects.
  - Example: erythromycin causes elevated blood levels of theophylline, which results in theophylline toxicity.
  - Other drugs or foods, such as grapefruit juice, can inhibit the activity of the CYP isoforms resulting in a higher than usual blood level of drugs metabolized by the P-450 system.

Plasma Protein Binding

- Protein binding can enhance or detract from a drug's performance.
- As a general rule, agents that are *minimally* protein bound penetrate tissues better, but are excreted much more rapidly.
- Drugs may bind to a wide variety of plasma proteins, including albumin.
- The concentration of several plasma proteins can be altered by many factors including stress, surgery, liver or kidney dysfunction, inadequate nutrition, and pregnancy.
- Drugs bound to plasma proteins will not enter the liver readily to be metabolized or excreted, resulting in a longer drug half-life and elevated blood levels in the elderly whose plasma albumin contents are lower.
  - Example: benzodiazepines can cause increased sedation and respiratory depression in the elderly.

Biotransformation

- The process that changes a drug to a different form that typically is more water-soluble.

Pathology

- Liver disease generally results in elevated levels of nonmetabolized drugs.

Absorption

- The route/initial process of the drug entering the body.
  - Gastrointestinal tract.
    - Oral ingestion.
    - Rectal (suppository).
  - Respiratory (inhaled medication into lungs, often via an inhaler).
  - Vascular (IV).
  - Skin (subcutaneous/intradermal).
  - Muscle (IM).

Excretion/Elimination

- The metabolized form of many drugs is more likely to stay in fluids and less likely to be reabsorbed by the kidney and back into the bloodstream.
- This facilitates excretion in urine.
- Elimination can also take place through the lungs, sweat, saliva, and feces.

Routes of Administration

- Oral.
  - Advantages:
    - Convenient access.
    - Painless route (no needles).
    - Economic—low cost.
  - Disadvantages:
    - Delayed onset (may take 30–45 minutes to show effect).
    - Unpredictable effects (same dosage may have different effects on different patients).
    - Patient compliance may be suboptimal (bad-tasting medications may be rejected by younger patients).
    - Difficult route of administration for patients with nausea.
- Topical.
  - Mucous membrane (e.g., topical anesthesia in dentistry).
  - Skin (e.g., nicotine patch).
  - Advantages:
    - Easily accessible.
    - More rapid absorption than via oral route.
    - Drugs enter systemic circulation without hepatic first pass.
  - Disadvantages:
    - Patient cooperation (patient might remove medication patch).
    - Slow onset.
    - Unpredictable effects.
    - Most drugs are poorly absorbed by this route.
- Intranasal: direct delivery to the brain may be facilitated by the incomplete blood–brain barrier in the olfactory region.
  - Advantages:
    - Rapid absorption.
    - Relatively minimal irritation.
    - Usually well tolerated by most patients.
    - Easily administered.
  - Disadvantages:
    - Patient cooperation could be an issue (pediatric patients).
    - Contraindicated for use in patients with upper respiratory infections.

Injection Routes

- Intramuscular (IM).
  - Advantages:
    - Good absorption due to vascularity of the muscle mass.
    - Easy access regardless of patient age, size, or nausea.
  - Disadvantages:
    - Variable and unpredictable onset of the drug effect.
    - Cannot titrate drug dosage.
    - Some drugs can be irritating to the muscle.
- Intravenous (IV).
  - Advantages:
    - Accurate dosage control.
    - Rapid onset.
    - Greater maximum volume of administration.
    - Greater dilution of the drug in normal saline or lactated Ringer's solution.
  - Disadvantages:
    - Greater potential for complications including infection and damage of the vasculature.
    - Greater discomfort associated with exploration and puncture of a subsurface vessel.
    - Increased technique sensitivity.

Inhalational Anesthesia

- Advantages:
  - Easily administered by trained professionals.
  - Painless.
  - Easily titrated.
  - Notable compliance for anesthesia in children.
  - Rapid absorption into systemic circulation through the lungs.
  - Most inhalational agents are general anesthetics except nitrous oxide.
- Disadvantages:
  - Special equipment required.
  - Inhalational general anesthetics may require intubation and ventilatory support.

Anesthetic Techniques

- Local anesthesia.
- Oral and nasal sedation.
- IM injection.

- Inhalation sedation (including nitrous oxide).
- IV mild/moderate sedation.
- IV deep sedation.
- General anesthesia.

Medications Utilized in Anesthesia/Sedation for Dental Patients

- Benzodiazepines.
  - Anxiolytic.
  - Anticonvulsant.
  - Antispasmodic.
  - Sedative/hypnotic.
  - Amnesic (anterograde amnesia).
  - Enhances the binding of gamma-aminobutyric acid (GABA) to the GABA receptor complex.
    - Increases frequency of chloride channel opening, which decreases the intracellular voltage and thus decreases neuronal firing.
  - Often available in both oral (PO) and IV forms.
  - Short-acting (< 6 hours) agents:
    - Triazolam (Halcion®) PO.
    - Midazolam (Versed®) PO, IV.
  - Intermediate (6–10 hours) agent:
    - Alprazolam (Xanax®) PO.
  - Long-acting (> 10 hours) agents:
    - Diazepam (Valium®) PO, IV.
    - Lorazepam (Ativan®) PO, IV.
  - Diazepam (Valium®).
    - Reduces anxiety.
    - Relaxes patient.
    - Dose-dependent anterograde amnesia.
    - Dose: 2–20 mg IV.
    - Easy to titrate.
    - Sedation effects may be reversed with flumazenil.
    - Insoluble in water.
    - Dissolved in propylene glycol which can cause vein irritation (phlebitis).
    - Half-life 20 to 40 hours.
  - Midazolam (Versed®).
    - Produces greater sedation than diazepam.
    - More profound anterograde amnesia than diazepam.
    - Shorter acting than diazepam.
    - Water soluble—less risk of thrombophlebitis than diazepam.

- ○ Dose: 1 to 5 mg IV.
- ○ Half-life: 1 to 4 hours.
- ○ Sedation effects may be reversed with flumazenil.
- Reversal agent for benzodiazepines.
  - Flumazenil (Romazicon®).
    - ○ Used to reverse the effects of benzodiazepines.
    - ○ Competitive antagonist at the GABA receptor.
    - ○ Dose: 0.2 to 1.0 mg IV.
    - ○ Reverses sedation and respiratory depression.
    - ○ Rapid onset (1–2 minutes).
    - ○ Patients might need to be observed for up to 2 hours because of the relatively short-term effects of flumazenil.
    - ○ Watch for resedation.
- Opioids.
  - Narcotics.
  - All are potent analgesics.
  - Act as agonist on mu, delta, kappa, and sigma receptors in the central nervous system (CNS).
  - Mu receptors (supraspinal).
    - ○ Responsible for analgesia and euphoria.
  - Available in both oral (PO) and IV forms.
    - ○ Fentanyl (IV, PO).
    - ○ Morphine (IV, PO).
    - ○ Codeine (PO).
    - ○ Meperidine (IV, PO).
  - Adverse effects:
    - ○ Pruritis (due to histamine release).
    - ○ Nausea/vomiting.
    - ○ Urinary retention.
    - ○ Constipation.
    - ○ Miosis.
    - ○ Respiratory depression.
  - Signs of opioid withdrawal:
    - ○ Hypertension.
    - ○ Piloerection ("goose bumps").
    - ○ Chills.
    - ○ Sweating.
    - ○ Nausea/vomiting.
    - ○ Abdominal cramping.
    - ○ Restlessness.
    - ○ Mydriasis.
    - ○ Lacrimation and rhinorrhea.
    - ○ Insomnia.

- o Manifestations not life-threatening unlike alcohol or benzodiazepine withdrawals.
- – All are respiratory depressants.
- – Minimal cardiovascular effects at normal doses.
- – Relieve pain without altering other senses (e.g., vision, hearing, touch).
- – All are reversible with naloxone (Narcan®).
- – Fentanyl.
  - o Synthetically modified morphine that is 100 times more potent.
  - o Rapid onset (< 1 minute).
  - o Short duration (30–60 minutes).
  - o Cardiovascular system remains stable, but may see bradycardia.
  - o No histamine release.
  - o Best narcotic for asthmatic patients and patients with a history of nausea and vomiting.
  - o Dose: 0.025 to 0.1 mg IV (25-100 µg).
  - o Can cause profound respiratory depression with deeper but infrequent breaths.
  - o Can cause chest wall rigidity if the administered dose is too potent and rapid.
  - o Most commonly used in current practice.
- – Morphine.
  - o A natural opioid.
  - o Narcotic analgesic standard—the standard to which other narcotics are compared.
  - o No longer commonly used for IV anesthesia in oral and maxillofacial surgery.
  - o Important emergency medication for myocardial infarction (dose 2–10 mg IV).
  - o High addiction potential.
- • Narcotic antagonist.
  - – Reverses the opioid's sedation and respiratory depression effects.
  - – Pure mu receptor antagonist.
    - o No opioid receptor agonist activity.
  - – Also reverses the opioid's analgesic effects.
    - o Can precipitate opioid withdrawal in patients with chronic pain on long-term opioids.
  - – Example: Naloxone (Narcan®).
    - o Dose: 0.4 to 2.0 mg IV.
    - o Rapid onset of action (1–2 minutes).
    - o Short duration of action (45 minutes).
    - o Patients may need to be observed for up to 2 hours following administration.

- Nitrous oxide/oxygen delivery system.
  - Must be capable of administering positive pressure oxygen.
  - Must have a scavenging system.
    - Two-tube system: (1) Scavenger tube removes exhaled nitrous oxide for the protection of the office staff. (2) Larger tube delivers nitrous oxide/oxygen gas mixture to patient.
- Oxygen.
  - Stored in green medical gas cylinder tanks of varying sizes.
  - Room air is approximately 21% oxygen.
  - Thirty percent or higher concentration of oxygen is recommended when delivering other pharmacologic agents to patients.
  - Recommended for all medical emergencies except hyperventilation (see Chapter 13, Management of Medical Emergencies).
  - May be used with all sedation cases.
  - Use with caution in patients with chronic obstructive pulmonary disease (COPD).
    - Flow should be no higher than 2 to 3 L/minute in patients with COPD.
- Nitrous oxide.
  - Indications for use:
    - Patients with mild apprehension undergoing dental procedures/extractions.
    - Anxious or hyperactive children.
  - Contraindications for use:
    - Absolute contraindications: (1) Pregnancy (may cause spontaneous abortion according to some studies, though controversial), (2) otitis media, (3) congenital pulmonary blebs, (4) sinus blockage, (5) bowel obstruction, (6) nasal obstruction, (7) cystic fibrosis, (8) COPD.
    - Relative contraindications: (1) Upper respiratory infection, (2) severe dental fear or anxiety, (3) patients with a prior bad experience or adverse reaction to nitrous oxide.
    - Asthma is not a contraindication for use of nitrous oxide.
  - Stored in blue medical gas cylinder tanks of varying sizes.
  - Is known by many as "laughing gas."
  - Physiology of nitrous oxide:
    - Acts on the CNS.
    - Produces a generalized neurologic depression and inhibits mental focus.
    - Decreases all forms of sensory input.
  - Solubility of nitrous oxide:
    - Relatively insoluble in blood.
    - Requires high alveolar concentration to achieve its intended effects.
  - Concentration effect:
    - The higher the concentration of nitrous oxide inhaled, the more rapid the increase in arterial concentration.

- Minimum of 30% oxygen delivery is required.
- Most flowmeters allow delivery of 30 to 70% nitrous oxide concentrations.
- Weak anesthetic.
- Provides analgesia.
- Produces euphoria and relaxation.
- No biotransformation.
- Side effects include:
  ○ Headaches.
  ○ Nausea/vomiting.
  ○ Lethargy.
  ○ Diffusion hypoxia.
- Diffusion hypoxia:
  ○ May occur if the patient is permitted to recover from nitrous oxide sedation while breathing in only room air.
  ○ Nitrous oxide from the bloodstream diffuses into the alveoli in the lungs diluting the oxygen concentration in the alveoli more rapidly than it can be replaced.
  ○ This causes decreased oxygen blood saturation, resulting in hypoxia.
  ○ Preventable via administration of high-concentration oxygen (100%) for at least 5 minutes during the recovery from nitrous oxide sedation. (1) 100% oxygen is almost five times more concentrated than the oxygen in room air (21%). (2) Allows for maintenance of adequate oxygen concentration in the alveoli.
- Complications of prolonged exposure to nitrous oxide:
  ○ Bone marrow suppression.
  ○ Megaloblastic anemia.
  ○ Leukopenia (low white blood cell numbers).
  ○ Neurological deficiencies: peripheral neuropathies.
  ○ Pernicious anemia.
- Nonflammable gas.
- May induce slight respiratory and myocardial depression.
- Patients with obstructive sleep apnea are sensitive to nitrous oxide and may benefit from lower concentrations of nitrous oxide.
- Not contraindicated for use in patients with asthma.
- Slight odor.
- Quick recovery once the gas has been discontinued.
• Technique for use of nitrous oxide:
  - Give verbal instructions prior to initiating nitrous oxide.
  - Confirm that female patients are not pregnant.
  - Inform patients that they "may feel like they are floating."
  - Inform patients that they "may feel tingling in their fingers and toes."
  - Total flow of air needed ≈ 6 to 8 L per minute typically.

- Respiratory minute ventilation = tidal volume (amount of air per breath) × respiratory rate (usual is 12–16 breaths per minute).
- Onset of effect is usually 2 to 3 minutes after initiating flow of nitrous oxide.
- *Low level* nitrous oxide administration is usually sufficient for children.
  - Thirty-three percent nitrous oxide: 2 L per minute nitrous oxide: 4 L per minute oxygen.
- *Medium level* nitrous oxide administration is usually sufficient for most adults; maximum dose recommended for children.
  - Fifty percent nitrous oxide: 3 L per minute nitrous oxide: 3 L per minute oxygen.
- *High level* nitrous oxide administration (for certain adults who are unaffected at medium level).
  - 62.5% nitrous oxide: 5 L per minute nitrous oxide: 3 L per minute oxygen.
- *Maximum level* nitrous oxide administration (for certain adults who are unaffected at high level).
  - Seventy percent nitrous oxide: 7 L per minute nitrous oxide: 3 L per minute oxygen.
- Procedure of administering nitrous oxide:
  - Place monitors: (1) Pulse oximeter—continuous, (2) blood pressure cuff set to every 5 to 10 minutes.
  - Apply shaded protective eyewear to patient.
  - Turn down brightness of ambient room lights.
  - Turn on pleasant music to drown out office noise.
  - Turn flowmeter on to 6 to 8 L per minute oxygen (100%) before placing the nasal hood on the patient.
  - Place the nasal hood on the patient ensuring that the size is appropriate and the fit is snug: (1) The patient should not feel air outflow on his/her eyes. (2) The patient should feel that he/she is getting enough air solely by breathing through their nose and nasal hood.
  - Ensure the scavenging system is turned on.
  - Slowly initiate administering nitrous oxide by incrementally adjusting the nitrous oxide dial on the flowmeter: (1) Allow 2 to 3 minutes to take effect. (2) If the nitrous oxide level is too low, the patient will not experience the relaxant effects. (3) If the nitrous oxide level is too high, the patient may experience nausea, dysphoria, sleepiness, disorientation, or sweating.
  - When the procedure is completed, turn off the nitrous oxide dial on the flowmeter and allow the patient to breathe 100% oxygen (6–8 L per minute) for at least 5 minutes: (1) This will prevent diffusion hypoxia and headache. (2) There is no need to slowly titrate down the nitrous oxide level when the procedure is completed.
- Oxygen flow must be maintained at least at 3 L per minute.
- If the oxygen tank is empty or the tubing is not properly connected, the nitrous oxide will shut off (*fail-safe mechanism*).

– If the nitrous oxide tank is empty or the tubing is not properly connected, the oxygen will keep running (as long as there is oxygen in the tank).

Other Adjunctive Medications Often Used in Sedation in Dentistry

- Anticholinergic agents/antisialogogues.
  - Decrease salivary, bronchial, and gastric secretions.
  - Examples include:
    - Atropine.
    - Glycopyrrolate (Robinul®).
  - Glycopyrrolate (Robinul®):
    - Twice as potent an antisialogogue (drying agent) as atropine.
    - Dose: 0.1 to 0.2 mg IV.
    - Produces less tachycardia than atropine.
- Antihistamines and ataractics.
  - Examples include:
    - Diphenhydramine (Benadryl®)—antihistamine.
    - Hydroxyzine (Vistaril®)—ataractic ("calming" drug).
  - Diphenhydramine (Benadryl®):
    - Good sedative properties.
    - Antiemetic properties.
    - Has an antisialogogue (drying) effect.
    - Used in treatment of allergic reactions.
    - Dose: 25 to 50 mg IV/PO.
  - Hydroxyzine (Vistaril®, Atarax®).
    - Sedative effects—frequently used for oral sedation in pediatric patients.
    - Potentiates narcotics and barbiturates.
- Corticosteroids.
  - Decrease swelling and inflammation.
  - Depress immune system.
  - Increase blood glucose.
  - Requires caution in patients with infections, ulcers, depression, tuberculosis, or preexisting immunosuppression.
  - Examples include:
    - Dexamethasone (Decadron®).
    - Hydrocortisone (Solu-Cortef®).
    - Methylprednisolone (Solu-Medrol®).
  - Dexamethasone (Decadron®):
    - Stabilizes cell membranes.
    - Minimizes swelling.
    - Dose: 4 to 20 mg IV.

Local Anesthetics in Dentistry

- Local anesthetics (LA).
  - Act on nerve fibers by altering the permeability of the nerve membrane to ions.
  - Prevent conduction of painful impulses.
  - Transient and reversible loss of sensation.
    - Once injected into tissue, LAs exists in both ionized and nonionized forms.
    - The nonionized base is able to readily penetrate many layers of tissue.
    - The base passes through the lipid nerve sheath and membrane.
    - Re-equilibration between the ionized and nonionized forms occurs once this passage is completed.
    - Once in the nerve axon, the ionized form is able to block sodium channels, prevent the inflow of sodium, slow the rate of depolarization, and thus prevent an action potential from occurring.
  - All LAs are composed of a lipophilic aromatic ring linked to a hydrophilic amino group.
  - This link is either an ester or an amide bond and determines classification (esters or amides).
  - The LA's lipophilic aromatic ring facilitates passage through the nerve sheath and membrane.
- Esters.
  - Metabolized by plasma pseudocholinesterases within the nearby blood.
  - Examples include:
    - Benzocaine.
    - Tetracaine.
    - Procaine (Novocaine®): (1) Infrequently used today due to the high incidence of allergic reactions. (2) May be used as an alternative for patients allergic to amide anesthetics.
- Amides.
  - Metabolized by the microsomal P-450 enzymes of the liver.
    - N-dealkylation.
    - Hydroxylation.
  - Examples include:
    - Lidocaine (Xylocaine®).
    - Mepivacaine (Carbocaine®).
    - Prilocaine (Citanest®).
    - Bupivacaine (Marcaine®).
    - Articaine (Septocaine®)—contains both an amide and an ester link, but is classified as an amide.
  - Amides generally have the letter "i" plus "caine" in their drug names (e.g., lido**caine**, mepiva**caine**, bupiva**caine**, prilo**caine**, art**icaine**).
  - The amides are longer lasting, less allergenic, and more effective than esters.

181

- Maximum dose of lidocaine with 1:100,000 epinephrine in adults is 7 mg/kg.
- An average adult should not receive more than 500 mg or about 10 to 11 cartridges.
  - Limited by maximum safe dose of epinephrine, which is approximately 0.2 mg.
- Lidocaine (Xylocaine®).
  - Relatively short duration of action.
  - Used with or without vasoconstrictors.
  - Epinephrine 1:50,000–1:200,000 concentration range.
  - Lidocaine is metabolized by the liver (both 'lidocaine' and 'liver' begin with "li").
  - The most common LA used in dentistry.
- Mepivacaine (Carbocaine®).
  - Longer duration of action than lidocaine, but often marketed in plain form without epinephrine.
  - Used with or without vasoconstrictors.
  - Neocobefrin 1:20,000.
- Prilocaine (Citanest®).
  - Ultra-short duration of action—without vasoconstrictor.
  - Long-acting—with vasoconstrictor.
- Bupivacaine (Marcaine®).
  - Long onset of action.
  - Long duration of action (6–8 hours).
  - Used with epinephrine (1:200,000).
  - Less profound anesthesia.
- Articaine (Septocaine®).
  - Intermediate-acting LA.
  - Four percent solution with 1:100,000 epinephrine.
  - Maximum dose ~ 7 carpules in the average adult patient.
  - The carpule stopper is latex-free.
  - Possibly linked to nerve injuries if given as a regional block in an area adjacent to a major nerve (inferior alveolar nerve, mental nerve, etc.).
- ▶ Table 10.1 lists the adult dosages for commonly used local anesthetics based on an average patient weight of 150 lbs.

Table 10.1 Dosages (adult) for local anesthetics (based on average weight of 150 lb)

Agent	mg/Carpule	Max dose (mg/kg)	Max dose (mg)
2% lidocaine	34	4.5	300
2% lidocaine with 1:100k epi	34	7	500
3% mepivacaine	51	6.6	400
0.5% bupivacaine with 1:200k epi	8.5	1.3	90
4% articaine with 1:100k epi	68	7	500

Table 10.2 Properties of local anesthetics

Agent	Lipid solubility	Protein binding	Duration	pKa	Onset time
Mepivacaine	1	75	Medium	7.6	Fast
Lidocaine	4	65	Medium	7.7	Fast
Bupivacaine	28	95	Long	8.1	Moderate

- ▶ Table 10.2 describes several important properties of commonly used local anesthetics.
  - Potency is determined by lipid solubility.
  - Greater lipid solubility produces a more potent LA because of rapid infiltration into the nerve cells (bupivacaine > lidocaine > mepivacaine).
  - Duration is determined by protein binding.
  - Greater protein binding creates a longer duration (bupivacaine > mepivacaine > lidocaine) by preventing excretion with fluids.
  - Onset time is determined by pKa.
  - The closer the pKa of a LA is to the pH of tissue (7.4), the more rapid the onset (mepivacaine > lidocaine > bupivacaine)
  - The pKa is the pH at which equal concentrations of ionized and nonionized forms exist.
- Vasoconstrictors.
  - Added to LAs to:
    ○ Increase duration of action of the anesthetic by constricting the movement of fluids and reducing anesthetic dispersion from the local area.
    ○ Make the anesthesia more profound.
    ○ Decrease rate of absorption of the anesthetic into the other organs and tissues of the systemic circulation.
    ○ Minimize systemic toxicity.
    ○ Encourage vasoconstriction which helps minimize surgical bleeding.
  - Epinephrine.
    ○ Sympathetic amine.
    ○ Increases heart rate and blood pressure.
    ○ Dilates bronchioles.
    ○ 1:50,000 to 1:200,000 concentration range.
    ○ 1:100,000 = 0.01 mg/mL (10 µg/mL).
  - NeoCobefrin.
    ○ Sympathetic amine.
    ○ Similar to epinephrine.
    ○ 1:20,000 concentration.
- ▶ Table 10.3 shows the duration of anesthesia with some commonly used local anesthetic agents.

Table 10.3 Duration of anesthesia with some local anesthetic agents

Local anesthetic agent	Maxillary infiltration		Inferior alveolar nerve block	
	Duration of pulpal anesthesia (min)	Duration of soft-tissue anesthesia (min)	Duration of pulpal anesthesia (min)	Duration of soft-tissue anesthesia (min)
Lidocaine 2% with 1:100,000 epinephrine[a]	45–60	170	85	190
Articaine 4% with 1:100,000 epinephrine [a]	45–60	190	90	230
Bupivacaine 0.5% with 1:200,000 epinephrine [a]	90	340	240	440
Prilocaine 4% plain	20	105	55	190
Mepivacaine 3% plain	25	90	40	165

[a]The duration of action is prolonged when combined with epinephrine, a vasoconstrictor. A "plain" solution contains no vasoconstrictive agent.
Source: From Baker EW. Anatomy for Dental Medicine, Second Edition. New York, Thieme ©2015.

Maximal safe doses of local anesthetics with vasoconstrictor

LIDOCAINE (2%)

- Maximal safe dose of lidocaine = 7.0 mg/kg
- 70 kg (average male) × 7.0 mg/kg = 490 mg
- 1 cartridge = 1.7cc (2% sol'n) = 34 mg/cart.
- 490 mg (total safe dose)/34 mg/cart. ≈ 14 cart.
- Safety factor of 30%: 14 cart. – 4 cart. = 10 cart.
- 70 kg × 2.2 lb/kg = 154 lb body weight
- 154 lb body weight/10 cart. ≈ 15 lb/cartridge

ARTICAINE (4%)

- Max. safe dose of articaine = 7.0 mg/kg
- 70 kg (average male) × 7.0 mg/kg = 490 mg
- 1 cartridge = 1.7cc (4% sol'n) = 68 mg/cart.
- 490 mg (total safe dose)/68 mg/cart. ≈ 7 cart.
- Safety factor of 15%: 7 cart. – 1 cart. = 6 cart.
- 70 kg × 2.2 lb/kg = 154 lb body weight
- 154 lb body weight/6 cart. ≈ 25 lb/cartridge

MEPIVACAINE (2%)

- Maximal safe dose of mepivacaine = 7.0 mg/kg
- 70 kg (average male) × 7.0 mg/kg = 490 mg
- 1 cartridge = 1.7cc (2% sol'n) = 34 mg/cart.
- 490 mg (total safe dose)/34 mg/cart. ≈ 14 cart.
- Safety factor of 30%: 14 cart. – 4 cart. = 10 cart.
- 70 kg × 2.2 lb/kg = 154 lb body weight
- 154 lb body weight/10 cart. ≈ 15 lb/cartridge

BUPIVACAINE (0.5%)

- Max. safe dose of mepivacaine = 2.0 mg/kg
- 70 kg (average male) × 2.0 mg/kg = 140 mg
- 1 cartridge = 1.8cc (0.5% sol'n) = 9 mg/cart.
- 140 mg (total safe dose)/9 mg/cart. ≈ 15 cart.
- Safety factor of 35%: 15 cart. – 5 cart. = 10 cart.
- 70 kg × 2.2 lb/kg = 154 lb body weight
- 154 lb body weight/10 cart. ≈ 15 lb/cartridge

Conversions and Calculations

- Drug concentration conversions:
  - How many milligrams (mg) per milliliter (mL) of drug are there in a 1% solution?
    - Concentration (%) = mg/mL.
    - Percent = per 100.
    - 1% solution = 1 g/100 mL.
    - 1 g = 1,000 mg
    - 1 g/100 mL = 1,000 mg/100 mL
    - 1,000 mg/100 mL = 10 mg/mL
  - Regarding epinephrine:
    - 1:100,000 = 1 g/100,000 mL
    - 1 g/100,000 mL = 1,000 mg/100,000 mL
    - 1,000 mg/100,000 mL = 1 mg/100 mL
    - 1 mg/100 mL = 0.01 mg/mL.
  - How many mL in a carpule?
    - 1.7 mL in each carpule of LA.
  - Example:
    - Lidocaine 2% solution = 20 mg/mL (1 carpule has 20 mg × 1.7 mL = 34 mg).
    - Epinephrine 1:100,000 = 0.01 mg/mL (1 carpule has 0.01 mg × 1.7 mL = 0.017 mg).

Complications of Local Anesthesia

- Toxicity.
  - Potential causes of toxicity:
    - Elevated plasma levels of LA.
    - Inadvertent intravascular injection of LA.
    - Violation of maximum milligram/kilogram (mg/kg) dose of LA.
  - Signs of LA toxicity:
    - Perioral/circumoral numbness—classic sign.
    - Initial signs (cardiovascular and CNS) – minimal to moderate overdose blood levels: (1) Tachycardia (elevated heart rate). (2) Hypertension (elevated blood pressure). (3) Tachypnea (elevated respiratory rate). (4) Drowsiness. (5) Confusion/slurred speech/stuttering. (6) Talkativeness/apprehension/excitedness. (7) Nystagmus. (8) Tinnitus (ringing in the ears). (9) Metallic taste.
    - Progressive signs—moderate overdose blood levels: tremors, hallucinations, hypotension, bradycardia, decreased cardiac output.
    - Advanced signs—moderate to high overdose blood levels: unconsciousness, generalized tonic–clonic seizures, ventricular dysrhythmias, respiratory and circulatory arrest.

- Allergy.
  - True hypersensitivity reactions to LA are rare.
  - Esters:
    - Derivatives of ρ-aminobenzoic acid (PABA).
    - More likely to induce allergic reactions than amides.
  - Methylparaben:
    - Bacteriostatic preservative.
    - May be the causative agent in many hypersensitivity reactions.
- Methemoglobinemia.
  - Hemoglobin is oxidized to methemoglobin.
  - Methemoglobin cannot bind and carry oxygen.
  - Caused by excessive doses of:
    - Benzocaine.
    - Prilocaine.
    - Lidocaine.
  - Clinical signs:
    - Decreased pulse oximetry.
    - Cyanosis.
    - Chocolate-colored blood visible in the surgical field.
- Treatment:
  - IV methylene blue (1–2 mg/kg of 1% solution over 5 minutes).
- Reversal of local anesthesia.
  - Phentolamine (OraVerse®) 1.7 mg in a 1.8 mL cartridge.
    - Short-acting alpha blocker.
    - Maximum dose is two cartridges.
    - Reverses vasoconstrictor effect and shortens LA duration.
    - Only for use with vasoconstrictor-containing LAs.
- Lidocaine toxicity.
  - Greatest risk for LA toxicity.
    - Geriatric and pediatric patients: Older patients metabolize drugs at a slower rate.
  - A geriatric patient who takes multiple medications may experience adverse drug reactions when lidocaine is administered.
    - Propranolol (Inderal®), a beta-adrenergic blocker, can reduce both hepatic blood flow and lidocaine clearance.
  - A possible additive adverse drug reaction exists with the administration of LAs and opioids in the geriatric and pediatric populations.
  - Opioids (fentanyl, meperidine, and morphine) may cause this amide LA additive effect because of their similar chemical structures (both are basic lipophilic amines) and a first-pass pulmonary effect.
  - The lungs may serve as a reservoir for these drugs with a subsequent release back into the system.

- ▶ Table 10.4 displays adult dosages for lidocaine as commonly used in oral and maxillofacial surgery practice.

Table 10.4 Adult dosages for lidocaine as commonly used in OMS practice

Agent	Cartridge size (mg)	Max dose[a] (mg/ kg)	Max dose[a] (mg/ lb)	Max dose[a] (mg)
2% lidocaine	34	4.5	2	300
2% lido w/ 1:100k epi	34	7	3.3	500

[a]Max dosages are based on an adult weight of 150 lb (or 70 kg) and taken from the manufacturer (Astra).

- Lidocaine toxicity and cardiovascular effects.
  - Lidocaine has a depressor effect on the myocardium.
  - Toxic doses of lidocaine cause sinus bradycardia because lidocaine increases the effective refractory period relative to the action potential duration and decreases cardiac automaticity.
  - If a very high dose has been administered, impaired cardiac contractibility, arteriolar dilation, and profound hypotension and circulatory collapse can result.
- Lidocaine toxicity and CNS effects.
  - Lidocaine usually has a sedative effect on the brain.
  - Initially, lidocaine toxicity depresses brain function in the form of drowsiness and slurred speech.
  - Symptoms can progress to unconsciousness and even coma.
- Risk factors for lidocaine toxicity.
  - Older age (> 60 years old) and pediatric patients.
  - Decreased body weight.
  - Congestive heart failure (CHF), acute myocardial infarction (MI).
  - Decreased hepatic function.
  - Concomitant use of drugs decreasing P-450 activity.
    - Cimetidine (Tagamet®): H_2 blocker that inhibits P-450, thereby allowing lidocaine to accumulate in the blood. This adverse reaction is seen only with cimetidine and not with other H_2 blockers.
    - A possible additive adverse drug reaction exists with administration of lidocaine and opioids in the geriatric and pediatric populations.
- Management of mild lidocaine overdose with rapid onset.
  - An overdose in which signs and symptoms develop within 5 to 10 minutes following drug administration is considered rapid in onset.
  - Possible causes include intravascular injection, unusually rapid absorption, or administration of too large a total dose.

- If clinical manifestations do not progress beyond mild CNS excitation and consciousness is retained, significant definitive care is not necessary.
- The LA undergoes redistribution and biotransformation, with the blood level falling below the overdose level in a relatively short time.
• ▶ Table 10.5 displays the most common forms of LA overdose.

Table 10.5 Most common form of LA overdose

Method of overdose	Likelihood of occurrence	Onset of signs and symptoms	Intensity of signs and symptoms	Duration	Primary prevention	Drug
Too large of a dose given	Most common	5–30 min	Gradual onset with increased intensity; may prove severe	Usually 5–30 min	Administer minimal doses	Amides; esters rarely

• Toxicity reversal.
  - Evidence suggests that the IV infusion of lipid emulsions can reverse the cardiac and neurologic effects of LA toxicity.
  - Case reports support the early use of lipid emulsion at the first sign of arrhythmia, prolonged seizure activity, or rapid progression of toxic manifestations in patients with suspected LA toxicity.
  - Intralipid 20% emulsion IV: administer 1 mL/kg over 1 minute.
  - Repeat twice more at 3- to 5-minute intervals.
  - Then (or sooner if stability is restored) convert to an infusion at a rate of 0.25 mL/kg/minute, continuing until hemodynamic stability is restored.
    ○ Increases proteins available for binding the LA.
  - As a last resort, can consider emergency hemodialysis.

Bibliography

[1] ACLS 2010 Guidelines. Circulation. 2010; 122 Suppl 3:S729
[2] Bursell B, Ratzan RM, Smally AJ. Lidocaine toxicity misinterpreted as a stroke. West J Emerg Med. 2009; 10(4):292–294
[3] Campagna JA, Miller KW, Forman SA. Mechanisms of actions of inhaled anesthetics. N Engl J Med. 2003; 348(21):2110–2124
[4] Malamed SF. Handbook of local anesthesia. 5th ed. St. Louis, Mosby, 2004
[5] Neal JM, Mulroy MF, Weinberg GL, American Society of Regional Anesthesia and Pain Medicine. American Society of Regional Anesthesia and Pain Medicine checklist for managing local anesthetic systemic toxicity: 2012 version. Reg Anesth Pain Med. 2012; 37(1):16–18

11 Management of Patients on Anticoagulants and Antiplatelet Medications

David R. Cummings, Jeffrey A. Elo, Alan S. Herford, Ho-Hyun Sun, Christopher H. Yi

Introduction

Anticoagulant and antiplatelet agents are prescribed to patients with histories or high probabilities of thromboembolic events (blood clots). These at-risk patients include those who have suffered from deep vein thrombosis, pulmonary embolism, or nonvalvular atrial fibrillation, an arrhythmia that predisposes patients to intracardiac clot formation.

Anticoagulants include the vitamin K antagonist warfarin (Coumadin®) and newer target-specific agents such as the direct thrombin inhibitor dabigatran (Pradaxa®) as well as factor Xa inhibitors apixaban (Eliquis®) and rivaroxaban (Xarelto®). Antiplatelet agents include clopidogrel (Plavix®), ticlopidine (Ticlid®), and aspirin. Adverse effects associated with these drugs can result in prolonged bleeding or bruising.

Dental providers must assess the risk of bleeding (hemorrhage) and clotting (thrombosis) in this patient population. Most patients undergoing oral surgery in the office do well and have uneventful courses with minimal blood loss. Significant blood loss during oral surgery is atypical, but such bleeding may prolong postoperatively as well.

A few simple steps can prevent bleeding complications and potentially dangerous postoperative sequelae. Practitioners must understand the patient's medical history, survey the patient's medications and note any potential interactions, understand the physiology of blood coagulation, evaluate the surgical site, remain aware of meticulous surgical techniques, and implement calm, sound clinical judgment.

Biology of Hemostasis

- There are two main phases of hemostasis:
  - Primary or cellular phase.
  - Secondary or humoral phase.

Primary (Cellular) Phase of Hemostasis

- Begins immediately after endothelial disruption and is characterized by vasoconstriction, platelet adhesion, and formation of a soft-tissue plug.

- Temporary local constriction of vascular smooth muscle; blood flow slows down.
- Within 20 seconds of injury, circulating von Willebrand factor attaches to the subepithelium at the injury site and adheres to the glycoproteins on the surface of the platelets.
- Platelets are then activated by contact with the collagen.
- Activated platelets then bind with circulating fibrinogen, forming a platelet plug.
- This is a short-lived phase of hemostasis and the plug can be easily dislodged.
- The soft platelet plug is stabilized during secondary hemostasis to form a clot.
- Vasoconstriction and reduction in blood flow are maintained by platelet secretion of serotonin, prostaglandin, and thromboxane as the coagulation cascade is initiated.
- If the patient has a disorder of primary hemostasis, there will be an abnormality in platelets.
  – Classic symptoms are:
    ○ Epistaxis (nose bleed).
    ○ Hemoptysis (coughing up blood).
    ○ Gastrointestinal (GI) bleeds.
    ○ Hematuria (blood in urine).
    ○ Menorrhagia (abnormal, prolonged menstruation).
    ○ Petechiae (< 3 mm).
    ○ Purpura (3–10 mm).
    ○ Ecchymoses (> 1 cm).
    ○ Easy bruising.
  – Specific pathologies can be divided into quantitative or qualitative platelet issues.

Secondary (Humoral) Phase of Hemostasis (▶ Fig. 11.1)

- Consists of the coagulation cascade.
- The end product of the cascade generates an active version of factor X which produces thrombin.
- Inactive factor X must be activated by:
  – Trauma that causes blood to leave the vessel (extrinsic pathway).
  – Damage to the inside of the vessel (intrinsic pathway).
- Goal is to stabilize the weak platelet plug.
- Factor X from the coagulation cascade generates thrombin from prothrombin.
- Thrombin converts fibrinogen in the platelet plug to fibrin.
- Fibrin is cross-linked to yield stable platelet-fibrin thrombus (blood clot) by factor XIII.

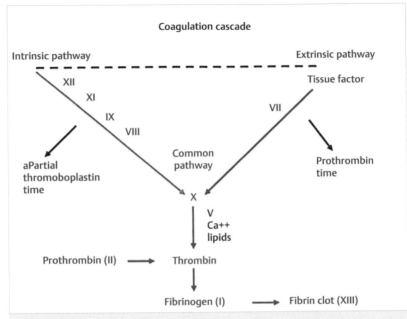

Fig. 11.1 Coagulation cascade demonstrating both the intrinsic and extrinsic pathways.

Clinical Pearls

- Partial thromboplastin time (PTT) measures the intrinsic pathway as well as the common pathway and is a better test for patients on heparin.
- Prothrombin time (PT) measures the extrinsic pathway as well as the common pathway and is a better test for patients on warfarin (Coumadin®).
- A Prothrombin Time test measures how quickly the patient's blood clots using a sample of the patient's blood.
- Prothrombin is a protein produced in the liver; it is one of many factors in the blood that promotes appropriate clotting.
- For patients receiving warfarin therapy, Prothrombin Time test results will be expressed as a ratio called the International Normalized Ratio.
- It is recommended that coagulation studies (PT and INR) be obtained within 1 day of surgery.
- Patients with an INR less than 4 can undergo dental extractions in an outpatient setting without discontinuation of their oral anticoagulation therapy.
- In healthy patients, an INR of 1.1 or below is considered normal.

Continued ▶

- An INR range of 2.0 – 3.0 is generally an effective therapeutic range for patients taking warfarin for disorders such as atrial fibrillation or a blood clot in the leg or lung.
- Patients with mechanical heart valves might need a higher INR.
- When the INR is higher than the recommended range, patients' blood clots more slowly than desired.

Disorders of the Coagulation Cascad (▶ Fig. 11.2)

- Due to factor abnormalities.
- Clinically present with deep tissue bleeding into muscles and joints with possible postoperative bleeding.
- Examples:
  - Hemophilia A (factor VIII deficiency).
  - Hemophilia B (factor IX deficiency).
  - von Willebrand disease (the most common inherited coagulation disorder, impairs platelet adhesion).
  - Vitamin K deficiency [occurs in newborns, long-term antibiotic users, as well as in patients with malabsorption issues (i.e., alcoholics), liver failure, and large volume blood transfusions].

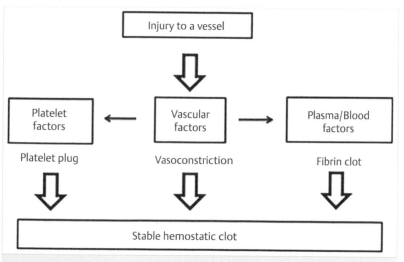

Fig. 11.2 Formation of a stable hemostatic clot following injury to a vessel requires various components all working together simultaneously.

Typical Patient—Discontinue or Keep on Anticoagulant Medications?

Table 11.1 Common categories and drug names for anticoagulant and antiplatelet medications

Anticoagulant/antiplatelet medications	
Drug class	**Drug names**
Anticoagulant	Warfarin (Coumadin®)
Antiplatelet agents	Clopidogrel (Plavix®)
	Ticlopidine (Ticlid®)
	Aspirin
Target-specific oral anticoagulants	Dabigatran (Pradaxa®)
	Rivaroxaban (Xarelto®)
	Apixaban (Eliquis®)

- ▶ Table 11.1 shows common categories and drug names for anticoagulant and antiplatelet medications.
- For a typical dental patient using anticoagulant or antiplatelet medications, there is no need to discontinue his or her regimen(s).
- Local hemostatic measures should be sufficient to control most of the bleeding.
- These measures include:
  - Mechanical pressure with gauze.
  - Hemostatic agents (e.g., Gelfoam® or Surgicel®).
  - Suturing.
  - Tranexamic acid mouthwash.

Medical Conditions with Higher Risks of Bleeding

- Age more than 65 years.
- Stroke (cerebrovascular accident).
- GI hemorrhage.
- Diabetes mellitus.
- Renal insufficiency.
- Recent myocardial infarction (MI).
- Anemia.
- History of significant bleeding in a prior surgery.
- Liver disease with synthetic dysfunction.
- Hematological (bleeding) disorder (von Willebrand disease, hemophilia, etc.).

Von Willebrand Disease

- Type 1: Most common and mildest form.
  - Responds to treatment with desmopressin (DDAVP).
- Type 2: Normal amounts of von Willebrand factor, but it does not work correctly.
  - Several types (types 2A, 2B, 2 M, 2N).
- Type 3: Most severe form of von Willebrand disease.
  - No von Willebrand factor present and low levels of factor VIII.

Treatment of Hemophilia

- Replacement of factor VIII for hemophilia A.
- Replacement of factor IX for hemophilia B.
  - Clotting factor concentrates can be made from pooled human blood.
  - Clotting factors can be made from recombinant clotting factors.

Maintaining Hemostasis

It is important to maintain hemostasis during surgery for several reasons:
- Improves visualization of the surgical field.
- Reduces surgical time.
- Decreases morbidity.
- Reduces need for blood product transfusions.

Several Factors can Contribute to Intraoperative Bleeding During Oral Surgery

- Absence of vasoconstrictor in local anesthetic.
- Tearing or puncturing of soft tissues.
- Exposed bone.
- Incision site position.
- Unseen sources of bleeding.
- Poor suturing techniques.
- Granulation tissue.
- Anticoagulant medications (aspirin, Plavix®, Coumadin®, etc.).
- Coagulopathies and platelet dysfunction.

Various Techniques Exist to Maintain Hemostasis in Oral Surgery

- Mechanical techniques.
- Thermal techniques.
- Chemical techniques.
- Topical hemostatics.
- Topical sealants and adhesives.

Mechanical Techniques to Maintain Hemostasis

- Direct pressure.
- Gauze.
- Sutures.
- Blood component/replacement therapy.

Thermal Techniques to Maintain Hemostasis

- Electrocautery.
- Hemostatic scalpel.
- Laser.

Chemical Techniques to Maintain Hemostasis

- Pharmacotherapy:
  - Epinephrine (vasoconstrictor in the local anesthetic).
  - Vitamin K (should only be ordered and supervised by the physician if the patient is taking warfarin (Coumadin®)).
  - Protamine (should only be ordered and supervised by the physician if the patient is taking heparin).
  - Aminocaproic acid.
  - Tranexamic acid (4.8% mouthwash).
  - Desmopressin (DDAVP) for type I von Willebrand disease.
  - Factor replacement for patients with hemophilia.

Topical Hemostatics to Maintain Hemostasis

- Collagen.
- Cellulose.
- Gelatins.
- Chitosan.
- Thrombin.

Collagen (Avitene®)

- Collagen-based products provide hemostasis through contact activation and the promotion of platelet aggregation which occurs as a direct reaction between blood and collagen.

Cellulose (Surgicel®)

- Cellulose-based products contain regenerated oxidized cellulose.
- They initiate clotting via contact activation, but the exact mechanism is not completely understood.

Gelatins (Gelfoam® sponge)

- Gelatin will conform to the wound and swell providing a tamponade effect in confined places.
- Clotting is initiated via contact activation.

Chitosan

- Chitosan bandages become extremely sticky when in contact with blood and form an adhesive-like seal.
- Chitosan has a positive charge and attracts the negatively-charged red blood cells forming a very tight seal or gel.

Thrombin

- First used in 1939 as a hemostatic agent.
- Its antigenicity was reported some time after.
- Widely used in topical applications.
- Clinical implications of induced antibodies is unclear.

Topical Sealants and Adhesives

- Fibrin sealants (Tisseel®).
- Synthetic glues (GluStitch® PeriAcryl).

Active and Passive Hemostasis

Active	Passive	Tissue sealants
Thrombin	Collagens	Fibrin sealants
	Cellulose	Polyethylene glycol
	Gelatins	Albumin/glue

Tranexamic Acid

- An antifibrinolytic that competitively inhibits the activation of plasminogen to plasmin, a molecule responsible for the degradation of fibrin.
- Fibrin forms the primary framework of blood clots.
- Used for modification of oral anticoagulants.
- Use of a 4.8% mouthwash in patients with INR of 2.0–4.0.
- Controls local antifibrinolytic activity.

Aminocaproic Acid (Amicar®)

- Derivative and analogue of the amino acid lysine.
- Effective inhibitor for enzymes causing fibrinolysis, which includes plasmin.
- Used for modification of oral anticoagulants.
- May be used as a mouthwash (2.5 grams per 10 mL).
- Swish gently over site for 2 minutes, then spit or swallow; repeat four times daily.
- May also be used in the syrup form.
- Contraindicated in patients with factor IX complex concentrates.
- ▶ Table 11.2 describes several common local hemostatic agents approved for use in oral and maxillofacial surgery.

Table 11.2 Common local hemostatic agents approved for use in oral and maxillofacial surgery

Local agent	Description	Features
Gelfoam®	Gelatin sponge, absorbs in 3–5 days	Addition of topical thrombin improves efficacy
Surgicel®	Oxidized regenerated cellulose, expands on contact with blood	Thrombin ineffective with this agent due to pH factors
Avitene®	Microfibrillar collagen, attracts platelets, stimulates aggregation	Thrombin ineffective with this due to pH factors, useful in moderate-severe bleeding
CollaCote® CollaTape® CollaPlug®	Collagen-based agent, matrix for coagulation cascade	Can be shaped to fit needs, absorbs in 10–14 days, useful in moderate-severe bleeding
Cyklokapron®	Tranexamic acid, inhibits conversion of plasminogen to plasmin	Hemostatic efficacy as postoperative mouth rinse
HemCon® Dental Dressing	Chitosan-based agent, electrostatic attraction between red blood cells, platelets and dressing	Early studies have suggested that it outperforms gauze pressure, collagen
Recothrom®	Topical thrombin, converts fibrinogen to fibrin	Useful with Gelfoam® and in moderate-severe bleeding

Drugs that Affect Platelet Function

- Antibiotics:
  - Long-term use kills off gut flora that produce vitamin K, which is essential for proper coagulation.
  - Vitamin K is used to gamma-carboxylate coagulation cascade factors II, VII, IX, X, and protein C and S.
  - Penicillin.
  - Cephalosporins.
- Antidepressants:
  - Mild inhibitory effect with platelets.
- Cardiovascular medications:
  - Propranolol: Decreases platelet responsiveness by a direct action on the platelet membrane, possibly by interfering with calcium availability. Platelet aggregation and basal cAMP level are influenced by beta-blockers in proportion to their affinity to different beta-adrenoceptors.
  - Verapamil: Inhibits platelet aggregation induced by threshold amounts of adenosine diphosphate (ADP), arachidonic acid (AA), and epinephrine. It also inhibits platelet adenosine triphosphate (ATP) release induced by AA and ADP.
- Food/food additives:
  - Ethanol.
  - Onions.
- Oncologic medications:
  - Many of the chemotherapeutic medications interfere with platelet function.

Commonly Prescribed Drugs that can Cause Bleeding

- Apixaban (Eliquis®).
- Aspirin (irreversibly inactivates cyclooxygenase).
- Citalopram (Celexa®).
- Clopidogrel (Plavix®).
- Dabigatran (Pradaxa®).
- Diclofenac (Voltaren®).
- Escitalopram (Lexapro®).
- Fluoxetine (Prozac®).
- Fluvoxamine (Luvox®).
- Ibuprofen.
- Ketoprofen.
- Ketorolac (Toradol®).

- Meloxicam (Mobic®).
- Nabumetone (Relafen®).
- Naproxen (Aleve®, Midol®).
- Paroxetine (Paxil®).
- Piroxicam (Feldene®).
- Rivaroxaban (Xarelto®).
- Sertraline (Zoloft®).
- Sulindac.
- Tenoxicam.
- Ticlopidine (Ticlid®).
- Warfarin (Coumadin®).

Herbal Drugs that can Cause Bleeding

- Ginkgo biloba.
- Garlic (in large amounts).
- Ginger.
- Ginseng.
- Feverfew.
- Saw palmetto.
- Willow bark.

Patients with Higher Risk of Bleeding—Management Considerations (▶ Fig. 11.3)

- For routine extractions, practitioners can safely and effectively provide care to patients taking anticoagulants after consultation with the patient's treating physician.
- For patients on warfarin, coagulation studies PT and INR should be obtained within 1 day of surgery.
- Patients with an INR of less than 4 can undergo extractions in an outpatient setting without discontinuation of their oral anticoagulation therapy.
- The extraction sites should be treated with resorbable gelatin sponges or other local coagulation techniques held in place with figure-8 suture closures.
- For patients requiring more-invasive surgery (e.g., large tori removal, trauma), the options include discontinuing warfarin and using heparin or low-molecular-weight heparin (Lovenox®) as bridging therapy, or maintaining the INR at 1.5 to 2.0.
- Patients taking antiplatelet therapy who require invasive/extensive oral surgery can be treated with single-drug therapy (instead of dual-drug

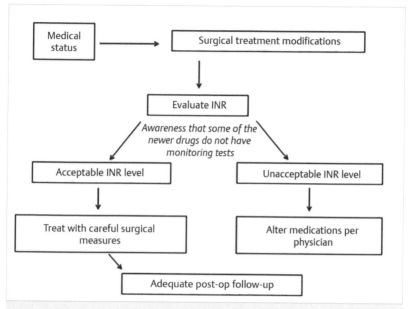

Fig. 11.3 Treatment algorithm for managing patients on warfarin (Coumadin®) who are in need of oral surgical procedures.

therapy, if they are currently on two antiplatelet medications) and the use of local measures for hemostasis.

- Alternatively, they can be treated with aspirin alone if they are receiving two-drug therapy (aspirin and Plavix®).
- If intraoperative bleeding is a concern secondary to the risk stratification assigned to a particular patient, it would be prudent to discuss the completion of the work in successive surgical stages, which might provide a more reliable postoperative hemostatic result.
- If the decision is made by the patient's treating physician to stop warfarin (Coumadin®), coagulation status should return to near normal in approximately 4 to 5 days.
  – However, evidence suggests a potential rebound hypercoagulability effect.
- There have been several well-documented episodes of thromboembolic events where warfarin was discontinued for a dental procedure.
- Any modification to the patient's anticoagulant/antiplatelet regimen prior to dental surgery should be done in consultation with and according to the advice or order of the patient's physician.

- Without anticoagulant or antiplatelet medications, some patients are at higher risk for blood clot development, which could result in thromboembolism, stroke, or MI.
- Considerations for drug cessation of any duration require a careful balancing against the potential consequences of prolonged bleeding.
- Within the currently available evidence, the general consensus indicates that no change is required to the drug regimens of patients receiving the newer target-specific oral anticoagulants (i.e., dabigatran, rivaroxaban, or apixaban) before undergoing dental interventions as long as local antihemorrhagic measures are taken.
- Current guidelines dictate that doses of even the older anticoagulants (e.g., warfarin) and antiplatelet agents (e.g., clopidogrel, ticlopidine, and/or aspirin) should not be altered before most dental procedures.
- The risks of stopping or reducing these agents (i.e., thromboembolism, stroke, MI) far outweigh the consequences of prolonged bleeding which can typically be controlled with local measures.
- In patients with unusual or comorbid conditions or in those receiving other therapy that can severely compromise hemostasis, a detailed consultation with the primary care physician is required to determine whether care can be delivered safely outside of a hospital setting.
- Some acceptable drug modifications may entail postponing the timing of the daily dose of the anticoagulant until after the procedure, timing the dental intervention as much as possible after the last dose of anticoagulant, or temporarily interrupting drug therapy for 24 to 48 hours.

Bibliography

[1] Achneck HE, Sileshi B, Jamiolkowski RM, Albala DM, Shapiro ML, Lawson JH. A comprehensive review of topical hemostatic agents: efficacy and recommendations for use. Ann Surg. 2010; 251 (2):217–228

[2] Aframian DJ, Lalla RV, Peterson DE. Management of dental patients taking common hemostasis-altering medications. Oral Surg Oral Med Oral Pathol Oral Radiol Endod. 2007; 103 Suppl:45.e1–45.e11

[3] American Dental Association Science Institute. (2015, October 22). Oral health topics: anticoagulant and antiplatelet medications and dental procedures. http://www.ada.org/en/member-center/oral-health-topics/anticoagulant-antiplatelet-medications-and-dental- Accessed on February 15, 2018

[4] Douketis JD, Spyropoulos AC, Kaatz S, et al. BRIDGE Investigators. Perioperative bridging anticoagulation in patients with atrial fibrillation. N Engl J Med. 2015; 373(9):823–833

[5] Grines CL, Bonow RO, Casey DE, Jr, et al. American Heart Association, American College of Cardiology, Society for Cardiovascular Angiography and Interventions, American College of Surgeons, American Dental Association, American College of Physicians. Prevention of premature discontinuation of dual antiplatelet therapy in patients with coronary artery stents: a science advisory from the American Heart Association, American College of Cardiology, Society for Cardiovascular Angiography and Interventions, American College of Surgeons, and American Dental Association, with representation from the American College of Physicians. J Am Dent Assoc. 2007; 138(5):652–655

[6] Hirsh J, Fuster V, Ansell J, Halperin JL, American Heart Association, American College of Cardiology Foundation. American Heart Association/American College of Cardiology Foundation guide to warfarin therapy. Circulation. 2003; 107(12):1692–1711

[7] Jeske AH, Suchko GD, ADA Council on Scientific Affairs and Division of Science, Journal of the American Dental Association. Lack of a scientific basis for routine discontinuation of oral anticoagulation therapy before dental treatment. J Am Dent Assoc. 2003; 134(11):1492–1497

[8] Mehta J, Mehta P, Ostrowski N, Crews F. Effects of verapamil on platelet aggregation, ATP release and thromboxane generation. Thromb Res. 1983; 30(5):469–475

[9] Napeñas JJ, Oost FC, DeGroot A, et al. Review of postoperative bleeding risk in dental patients on antiplatelet therapy. Oral Surg Oral Med Oral Pathol Oral Radiol. 2013; 115(4):491–499

[10] Napeñas JJ, Hong CH, Brennan MT, Furney SL, Fox PC, Lockhart PB. The frequency of bleeding complications after invasive dental treatment in patients receiving single and dual antiplatelet therapy. J Am Dent Assoc. 2009; 140(6):690–695

[11] Steinberg BA, Peterson ED, Kim S, et al. Outcomes Registry for Better Informed Treatment of Atrial Fibrillation Investigators and Patients. Use and outcomes associated with bridging during anticoagulation interruptions in patients with atrial fibrillation: findings from the Outcomes Registry for Better Informed Treatment of Atrial Fibrillation (ORBIT-AF). Circulation. 2015; 131 (5):488–494

[12] Wahl MJ. Dental surgery in anticoagulated patients. Arch Intern Med. 1998; 158(15):1610–1616

[13] Winther K, Knudsen JB, Gormsen J, Jensen J. Effect of metoprolol and propranolol on platelet aggregation and cAMP level in hypertensive patients. Eur J Clin Pharmacol. 1986; 29(5):561–564

12 Hypertension Guidelines

Ronald Caloss, Jr., Jeffrey A. Elo, Alan S. Herford

Hypertension

- Approximately 75 million Americans suffer from hypertension (HTN).
- Both primary and secondary HTN are usually asymptomatic.
- Studies have shown a consistent correlation between elevated blood pressure (BP) and cardiovascular disease (CVD).
- End organ damage and microalbuminuria often accompany heart failure and may portend future severe events.
- Primary, or essential, hypertension occurs in more than 90% of case with no identifiable causes.
    - Its etiology likely involves both genetics as well as environmental factors that have been linked to sympathetic overactivity and altered renal transport.
- Secondary HTN occurs as an unwanted complication of other conditions such as obstructive sleep apnea, coarctation of the aorta, Cushing's disease, renal artery stenosis, hyperaldosteronism, pheochromocytoma, and hyperthyroidism.
- In November 2017, the medical community published new BP targets and treatment recommendations.
    - For years, HTN was classified as a BP reading of 140/90 mm Hg or higher, but the updated guideline classifies HTN as a BP reading of 130/80 mm Hg or higher.
    - The updated guideline also provides new treatment recommendations which include corrections to lifestyle changes as well as BP-lowering medication regimens.
- Dentist practitioners should be well informed of these new guidelines because many dental patients will be reporting changes to their medical and medication histories.
- The 2017 Hypertension Guideline changes the definition of HTN, which now includes any systolic BP measurement of 130 mm Hg or higher or any diastolic BP measurement of 80 mm Hg or higher (▶ Table 12.1).

Table 12.1 Classification of blood pressure (BP) in adults

BP category	Systolic BP (mm Hg)		Diastolic BP (mm Hg)
Normal	<120	and	<80
Elevated	120–129	and	<80
Hypertension			
Stage 1	130–139	or	80–89
Stage 2	≥140	or	≥90

Pharmacologic Recommendations

- The updated guideline recommends BP-lowering medications for stage 1 HTN patients with clinical CVD, patients with 10-year risk of atherosclerotic CVD (ASCVD) of 10% or greater, or for those with stage 2 HTN.
- For stage 2, the recommendation is two BP-lowering medications in addition to healthy lifestyle changes, which amounts to a more aggressive treatment standard.
  - Previous guidelines recommended starting patients on only one BP-lowering medication.
- The guideline also updates the recommendations for specific populations.
  - For example, because more patients of African descent have been diagnosed with HTN than other groups, two or more anti-HTN medications are recommended to achieve a target of BP less than 130/80 mm Hg.
  - Thiazide-type diuretics and/or calcium channel blockers are also indicated because of their increased efficacy in lowering BP alone or in multidrug regimens.
  - Morbidity and mortality attributed to HTN are more common in adults of African and Hispanic descent compared to predominantly European populations.
- Monthly physician follow-up is recommended for adults with a novel or adjusted HTN drug regimen in order to gauge proper response until their BP is under control.

Emphasis on Cardiovascular Disease

- The updated guideline provides recommendations for patients with clinical CVD and makes new recommendations for using the ASCVD risk calculator:
  - Use BP-lowering medication for **primary** prevention of CVD in adults with no history of CVD *and* an estimated 10-year ASCVD risk of less than 10% *and* a systolic BP of 140 mm Hg or greater *or* a diastolic BP of 90 mm Hg or greater.
  - Use BP-lowering medications for **secondary** prevention of recurrent CVD events in patients with clinical CVD *and* an average systolic BP of 130 mm Hg or greater or a diastolic BP of 80 mm Hg or greater *and* for **primary** prevention in adults with an estimated 10-year ASCVD risk of 10% or greater with an average systolic BP of 130 mm Hg or greater *or* average diastolic BP of 80 mm Hg or greater.

No Prehypertension

- The updated guideline eliminates the term *prehypertension* and instead uses the term *elevated BP* for a systolic BP of 120 to 129 mm Hg and a diastolic BP of less than 80 mm Hg.

More Hypertension Patients

- Because the new threshold for HTN is lower (130/80 mm Hg), more people will be diagnosed with the condition.
- However, most of these new patients can prevent HTN-related health problems through lifestyle changes alone.

Hypertensive Urgency Versus Hypertensive Emergency (▶ Table 12.2)

- Hypertensive urgency is associated with a severe BP elevation in an otherwise stable patient without acute or impending change in target organ function, i.e., no organ damage or dysfunction.

Table 12.2 Hypertensive crises: emergencies and urgencies

Hypertensive crises	Systolic BP (mm Hg)		Diastolic BP (mm Hg)	Treatment or follow-up
Hypertensive urgency	>180	and/or	>120	Many of these patients are noncompliant with anti-HTN therapy and do not have clinical or laboratory evidence of new or worsening target organ damage; reinstitute or intensify anti-HTN drug therapy, and treat anxiety as applicable
Hypertensive emergency	>180 + target organ damage	and/or	>120 + target organ damage	Admit patient to an intensive care unit for continuous monitoring of BP and parenteral administration of an appropriate agent in those with new/progressive or worsening target organ damage

Source: Whelton PK, Carey RM, Aronow WS, et al. ACC/AHA/AAPA/ABC/ACPM/AGS/APhA/ASH/ASPC/NMA/PCNA guideline for the prevention, detection, evaluation, and management of high blood pressure in adults: a report of the American College of Cardiology/American Heart Association Task Force on Clinical Practice Guidelines. Hypertension 2018;71:1269–1324. © 2017 American Heart Association.

- Hypertensive emergency is a severe elevation in BP associated with evidence of new or worsening target organ damage.
- Target organ dysfunction includes encephalopathy, cerebrovascular accident (CVA), myocardial infarction, congestive heart failure, pulmonary edema, angina, dissecting aneurysm, and eclampsia.
- The therapy is to reduce the BP by no more than 25% over 30 to 60 minutes, and then to 160/100 in 2 to 6 hours.
- The goal is to return BP to a level where autoregulation restores normal perfusion pressures to vital organs and not necessarily to normal BP.
- Excessive drops in pressure may precipitate ischemia.

Focus on Accurate Measurements

- To ensure accurate measurements, ensure the instrument in use is properly calibrated.
- The updated guideline also stresses on the basic processes for accurately measuring BP, including some simple yet critical actions before and during measurements.
- For accurate in-office measurements, consider the following:
  - Have the patient avoid tobacco, caffeine, or exercise within 30 minutes before measurements.
  - Have the patient empty his or her bladder.
  - Have the patient sit quietly for at least 5 minutes before measurements and remain still during measurements.
  - Support the limb used to measure BP, ensuring that the BP cuff is at heart level and that the cuff size is appropriate.
  - Avoid taking measurement over clothes.
  - Measure on both arms and use the higher reading.
  - An average of two to three measurements taken on two to three separate occasions will minimize error and provide a more accurate estimate.

Focus on Self-monitoring

- Because BP measured in-office is often higher than ambulatory or home BP, the updated guideline emphasizes having patients monitor BP on their own for HTN diagnosis, treatment, and management.
- Patients should:
  - Use the same validated instrument at the same time of day when taking at-home measurements to more accurately compare results.
  - Position themselves correctly, with the bottom of the cuff directly superior to the bend of the elbow.

- Optimally, take at least two readings 1 minute apart each morning before medication and each evening before supper.
- Obtain weekly readings 2 weeks after a treatment change and during the week before a clinic visit.
- Record all readings accurately.
- Use a monitor with built-in memory and bring it to all clinic appointments.
• For clinical decision-making, the patient's physician should consider patient's final BP as the average of two or more BP readings on different occasions.

Treatment Recommendations

• The updated guideline presents new treatment recommendations that include lifestyle changes as well as BP-lowering medications.
• ▶ Table 12.3 displays common hypertension medications that may be seen daily in dental clinical practice.

Table 12.3 Common hypertension medications

Type	Examples
Diuretics	Hydrochlorothiazide (HCTZ), furosemide, spironolactone, triamterene
Angiotensin-converting enzyme inhibitors (ACE inhibitors)	Lisinopril, captopril, enalapril, benazepril
Angiotensin receptor blockers (ARBs)	Losartan, valsartan, candesartan, irbesartan
Calcium channel blockers (CCBs)	Verapamil, diltiazem, dihydropyridine, nifedipine
Beta blockers	Atenolol, carvedilol, propranolol, metoprolol

• Lifestyle changes can reduce systolic BP by approximately 4 to 11 mm Hg for patients with HTN, with diet and exercise incurring the greatest benefit.
- In addition to promoting the Dietary Approaches to Stop Hypertension (DASH) diet, which is rich in fruits, vegetables, whole grains, and low-fat dairy products, the updated guideline recommends reducing sodium intake and increasing potassium intake to reduce BP.
- However, some patients—especially those with kidney disease or those requiring medications that react with certain ions—may be harmed by excess potassium.
- Each patient's ideal body weight is the best goal, but approximately 1 mm Hg BP reduction may be seen for every 1 kg reduction in body weight.
- Recommendations for physical activity include 90 to 150 minutes of aerobic and/or dynamic resistance exercise per week as well as three sessions per week of isometric resistance exercises.
- For patients who drink alcohol, aim for reducing alcohol intake to two or fewer drinks daily for men and no more than one drink daily for women.

New targets for comorbidities

- For patients with comorbidities, the updated guideline generally recommends prescribing BP-lowering medications in patients with clinical CVD and new stage 1 or stage 2 HTN to target a BP of less than 130/80 mm Hg (this was previously indicated at less than 140/90 mm Hg).
- The guideline recommends different follow-up intervals based on the stage of HTN, type of medication, level of BP control, and presence of target organ damage.

Dental Considerations for Managing Patients with Hypertension

Table 12.4 (Sample) Clinical protocol for patients with hypertension

Systolic pressure (mm Hg)	Diastolic pressure (mm Hg)	Dental treatment
≤ 139	≤ 89	No contraindications to elective dental treatment
140–159	90–99	Elective dental treatment okay. Monitor blood pressure during appointment
160–179	100–109	Emergency or noninvasive dental treatment only. Medical consultation prior to elective dental treatment is recommended
≥ 180	≥ 110	No dental treatment of any kind. Refer to Emergency Room. Call 911 if patient is symptomatic

- ▶ Table 12.4 suggests a sample clinical protocol for managing dental patients with hypertension.
- American Society of Anesthesiologists (ASA) Guidelines:
  - ASA II: 140 to 160/90 to 95 mm Hg
    - Manage with *stress reduction protocol*, which includes: (1) morning appointments; (2) short appointments (1 hour or less); (3) sedation, if patient is a candidate; (4) pain control (profound local anesthesia); (5) minimize patient wait time (waiting increases patient anxiety); (6) consider preprocedural sedative (oral benzodiazepine or nitrous oxide); (7) recognize signs of disease.
  - ASA III: 160 to 200/95 to 115 mm Hg
    - Manage with stress reduction protocol.
    - Consider physician consult to improve medical management prior to dental/surgical intervention.
  - ASA IV: > 200/ > 115 mm Hg
    - Elective dental treatment is NOT recommended.
- Minimize epinephrine (< 0.04 mg per appointment; approximately 2.2 carpules (1.7 mL each) of 2% lidocaine with 1:100k epinephrine).

Hypertensive Crisis

- Pathophysiology:
  - Markedly elevated BP constituting a hypertensive crisis usually occurs when there is excessive adrenergic or adrenaline-like stimulation.
  - This leads to vasoconstriction as well as increased rate and contractile force of the heart.
  - Precipitating factors can include pain, hypoxia, hypercarbia, and severe pulmonary or cardiovascular compromise (e.g., pulmonary edema).
    - Adrenal tumors such as pheochromocytoma may also rarely cause hypertensive episodes.
- Diagnosis:
  - Markedly increased BP, sometimes as high as 240 to 250 mm Hg (systolic) or 140 mm Hg and greater (diastolic).
- Position:
  - Semi-reclined.
- Treatment:
  - Before treatment is instituted, one should initially try to determine the cause (e.g., pain or hypoxia and hypercarbia).
  - If the cause can be determined, possible measures should be undertaken to correct the underlying cause.
  - If the BP remains elevated, it can be treated with an antiadrenergic agent such as labetalol or a vasodilator such as hydralazine.
  - Sequence of treatment:
    - Stop procedure; assure patient if he/she is conscious.
    - Assess pain control, oxygenate, and then monitor electrocardiograph to help determine etiology and concomitant conditions.
    - Treat cause, if possible.
    - If blood pressure does not return to acceptable levels within a few minutes, administer either: (1) *Nonasthmatic patient*: labetalol 5 to 20 mg intravenous (IV) over 2 min. Shorter-acting esmolol may also be used at a rate of 1 mg/kg IV, then 25 to 50 mg every 5 minutes as needed; (2) *Asthmatic patient without cardiovascular compromise*: Hydralazine 5 to 25 mg IV (watch for increased heart rate and decreased blood pressure).
    - Institute caution. Do not overtreat.

Stroke (Cerebrovascular Accident)

- Pathophysiology:
  - A stroke, or CVA, is an acute loss of circulation to a portion of the brain due to either occluded arteries or intracranial hemorrhage.

– When circulation to the affected area is lost, the patient develops neurologic symptoms such as paralysis, weakness, or loss of sensation on one side of the body.

- Diagnosis:
  – Altered consciousness, hemiparesis, hemiparalysis, aphasia, headache, blurred vision, or sudden HTN greater than 140/90 mm Hg.
- Position:
  – Comfortable, semi-upright.
- Treatment:
  – Although definitive treatment for stroke is beyond the scope of a dentist and his/her staff, early detection and transfer to a stroke treatment facility is essential to the patient's outcome.
  – A prehospital assessment such as the Cincinnati Prehospital Stroke Scale should be performed, the "ABCs" followed, and the patient should be transferred to the appropriate facility as soon as possible.
    ○ Check for facial droop upon smiling.
    ○ Monitor drifting of the arms when they are stretched forward for 10 seconds or more.
    ○ Note any speech slurring.
  – Sequence of treatment:
    ○ Terminate procedure, administer oxygen, activate EMS—call 911.
    ○ Airway, breathing, circulation ("ABCs").
    ○ IV access and fluid bolus if patient is hypotensive.
    ○ Facilitate transport to hospital/stroke center as soon as possible.

13 Management of Medical Emergencies

Brett J. King, Jeffrey A. Elo, Alan S. Herford

Introduction

This chapter provides important information for the dental practitioner to aid in the diagnosis and treatment of common medical emergencies encountered in dental practices utilizing commonly employed principles of prevention, organization, recognition, and stabilization.

There are four medical emergencies that occur most commonly in a dental practice setting. These are as follows:

- Syncope (*most common*).
- Allergy.
- Angina.
- Postural (orthostatic) hypotension.

These four emergencies constitute nearly 75% of all office-based medical emergencies.

Why Medical Emergencies Occur and How to Avoid Them

- Fear: Recognize that most patients do not enjoy visiting the dentist.
- Stress: Investigate strategies that will reduce patient stress (behavioral, pharmacologic).
- Allergies: Investigate adverse drug reactions and avoid using or prescribing these meds.
- Drug interactions: Develop a deeper understanding of commonly used medications in the dental office.
- Medically compromised patient:
  - Consult, when needed, with the patient's physician to develop best practices in managing these difficult patients.
  - Consider shorter morning appointments when patients might be feeling better.

How can the Dental Provider Prevent Medical Emergencies?

- Prevention:
  - Obtain a complete medical history.
  - Record and review patient's vital signs.

- Evaluate the current status of each of the patient's medical comorbidities.
    - Contact the patient's primary physician to further explore the current status of each of the patient's medical conditions.
- By evaluating the current status of each medical condition, the practitioner not only becomes more confident in managing the patient's dental problems but also takes steps for preventing medical emergencies in the dental office.
- A complete medical history is the foundation of investigating a patient's current health status.
- Record vital signs:
    - Blood pressure (BP).
    - Heart rate.
    - Respiratory rate.
    - Temperature.
    - BP should be recorded at each patient visit.
- A review of the patient's health history ought to be performed at each clinic visit to inquire about any changes in medical conditions, new diagnoses, medication changes, or new allergies.
    - Any updates should be noted in the patient's health record.

Vital Signs

- When recording vital signs, it is important to have the necessary equipment available.
    - BP cuff (sphygmomanometer) and stethoscope to record BP.
    - Finger palpation and a watch with a second hand to record heart rate.
    - Thermometer or temperature probe to record temperature.

Blood Pressure—Clinical Limitations

- It is important that each dental office have a clearly written and consistently enforced policy for dealing with elevated patient BPs.
- Patients with significantly elevated BP are at increased risk of a stroke or cardiac event.
- Blood pressure ≥ 180/110:
    - Defer elective treatment.
    - Patient should be referred to his/her physician as soon as possible for evaluation and management.
    - If the patient is symptomatic (headache, dizziness, confusion), 911 should be called, emergency medical response should be activated, and the patient should be transported via ambulance to the nearest emergency room or stroke center.
- Blood pressure ≥ 160/100 but < 180/110
    - May proceed cautiously with emergency/non-elective dental treatment if patient's elevated blood pressure is asymptomatic.

- Consider monitoring BP during the procedure with automated noninvasive BP monitor set at regular (5- or 10-minute intervals).
  - Refer patient to his/her physician for appointment within 1 month.
- Blood pressure ≥ 140/90 but < 160/100
  - Proceed with dental treatment, but encourage patient to see his/her physician for evaluation.
- Blood pressure < 120/80
  - No contraindications to elective dental treatment.
- Many patients have complex medical conditions and may be undergoing management with several medical doctors.
  - These patients pose challenges to dental providers, such as:
    - Potential for drug interactions if they are on several medications.
    - Patients may be elderly or more fragile and less likely to tolerate stress.
    - Carry a higher risk of undergoing a medical emergency.
- Dental providers should be prepared to cancel treatment or postpone treatment based on uncontrolled systemic diseases (BP too high, blood sugar too high or low) even if the patient insists that he/she is okay.
- The dental provider is ultimately responsible for managing the patient during dental treatment.
- If the dental provider is not comfortable, treatment should be canceled or postponed.

Stress Reduction to Prevent Medical Emergencies

- Alleviating patient fears is instrumental in preventing common medical emergencies in the dental office.
- Taking time to establish good rapport with patients is a worthwhile investment of time. This decreases patient anxiety as the patient feels more comfortable.
- Appropriate appointment times.
- Good communication with the patient before, during, and after the appointment/procedure.
- Profound local anesthesia/pain control.

Scheduling Appointments to Minimize Risk

- Certain patients may feel better at certain times of the day.
- Diabetic patients do better with morning appointments.
- Cardiac patients often feel better in the late morning/early afternoon.

Pain Control

- Administering profound local anesthesia in appropriate doses is critical for treatment success and helps minimize anxiety and discomfort during procedures.
- The proper use of effective sedation techniques can help patients tolerate dental procedures, but not every patient is a good candidate for sedation.
- Certain medical and emotional conditions can interfere with the ability of sedation techniques to be provided in a safe and effective manner.
- A clinician needs to be trained, licensed, and/or permitted to employ certain sedation techniques.
- Manage postoperative pain with appropriate prescriptions.
- Consider nitrous oxide or other sedation techniques, if appropriate.

Cardiopulmonary Resuscitation

- The first step when initiating cardiopulmonary resuscitation (CPR) is to establish unresponsiveness.
- ABCDs of CPR.
- Airway:
  - Head tilt.
  - Jaw thrust (if neck trauma suspected).
- Breathing:
  - Look for chest rise.
  - Listen for breath sounds.
  - Feel for chest rise.
  - If respirations are absent/inadequate, then provide rescue breathing.
    - Bag valve mask (BVM).
  - Ventilation rate: 1 breath every 5 to 6 seconds (10 to 12 breaths per minute).
- Circulation:
  - Check pulse.
  - If pulse is absent, then initiate chest compressions.
    - Compression-to-ventilation ratio is 30:2 (rate of 100 compressions per minute).
- Defibrillation:
  - Automated external defibrillator (AED).

215

Algorithms for the Management of Medical Emergencies

ACUTE ADRENAL INSUFFICIENCY

Pathophysiology

- The adrenal glands are located on top of the kidneys and produce corticosteroids and catecholamines.
- Corticosteroids provide resistance to stress, maintain vascular reactivity, increase plasma glucose, and control metabolism of carbohydrates, proteins, and fats.
- When exogenous corticosteroids are prescribed (e.g., prednisone), the glands begin decreasing output, become suppressed, and lose much of their ability to respond to stress.
- When the patient is exposed to a stressful situation such as surgery, the adrenal glands are unable to provide adequate corticosteroids to maintain vascular reactivity, and the BP falls.

Diagnosis

- Weakness, fatigue, and hypotension induced by surgical stress.
- Other symptoms include pallor, diaphoresis, nausea, tachycardia, and loss of consciousness.

Position

- Trendelenburg (supine, but with feet elevated above head).

Treatment

- The patient should be placed in the Trendelenburg position, intravenous fluids rapidly administered, and hydrocortisone given to augment the inadequate cortisol production of the adrenal glands.
- Sequence of treatment:
  - Terminate the procedure, activate Emergency Medical Services (EMS)—call 911.
  - Airway, breathing, circulation (ABCs).
  - Intravenous (IV) access if not already available.
    - Give rapid infusion of 5% dextrose with normal saline.
  - Hydrocortisone 100 mg IV or dexamethasone 4 mg IV.
  - Transport to a medical facility or an emergency room.

ACUTE CORONARY SYNDROME—ANGINA PECTORIS

Pathophysiology

- Angina is a crushing pain in the chest caused by blockage of the coronary arteries.
- The pain can radiate to areas such as the shoulder, neck, arms, or the mandible.
- In *stable* angina, the atheroma retains a relatively stable fibrous cap that prevents the accumulation of blood clot around it.
- The decreased lumen size leads to pain during times of exertion.
- In *unstable* angina, the atheroma may have a ruptured cap that attracts the accumulation of blood.
- Eventually, a blood clot forms at the site and the blood vessel becomes temporarily occluded at unpredictable time intervals.

Continued ▶

ACUTE CORONARY SYNDROME—ANGINA PECTORIS

- The occlusion of the artery reduces the blood flow, and therefore oxygen supply to the heart muscle which results in unpredictable angina or chest pain even during rest.
- Symptoms of both stable and unstable angina occur only when a coronary artery experiences occlusion of 70% or greater of its luminal area.
- Progressive occlusion of the coronary arteries leads to the "acute coronary syndrome."
- Angina is frequently the initial clinical manifestation of this syndrome.
- However, the occlusion may ultimately result in a myocardial infarction (MI).
- Hence, there is a continuum in the treatment approach ("ONAM"—oxygen, nitroglycerin, aspirin, morphine).

Diagnosis

- Vice-like, heavy, squeezing chest pain.
- Pain may radiate to shoulder, neck, arms, or jaw (mandible).

Position

- Semi-seated (semi-upright sitting position), loosen tight clothing for patient comfort.

Treatment

- The first steps in treatment consist of administering oxygen (O_2) as well sublingual nitroglycerin to dilate the coronary arteries, increase oxygen delivery, and improve blood flow.
- This helps decrease cardiac demand while increasing plasma oxygen supply to prevent infarction (death) of the myocardium (heart muscle).
- Sequence of treatment:
  - Terminate the procedure, pack surgical site, assure patient.
  - Activate EMS—call 911.
  - Administer O_2 via nasal mask or cannula at 4–5 L/minute of flow.
  - Constantly monitor vital signs.
  - Administer sublingual nitroglycerin (1–2 sprays or 1 tablet).
    - Repeat at 5-minute intervals for up to two doses.
  - If pain persists after 10 min of onset, assume that MI has occurred, administer morphine sulfate 1.5–3.0 mg/5 minutes, and treat as MI with a dose of aspirin 160–325 mg as well as additional morphine as needed.
  - Transport to hospital.

ACUTE CORONARY SYNDROME—MYOCARDIAL INFARCTION

Pathophysiology

- The acute coronary syndrome develops because of fatty deposits (atherosclerotic plaques) within the coronary artery walls.
- Eventually, this deposit may lose its capsular cover and a blood clot may form which permanently and completely occludes the artery.
- Subsequent ischemia leads to death or necrosis of the area of the myocardium supplied by the artery.

Diagnosis

- Usually heavy, squeezing chest pain that does not respond to nitroglycerin.

Continued ▶

ACUTE CORONARY SYNDROME—MYOCARDIAL INFARCTION

- Twenty percent of MI patients have no pain but exhibit nausea, vomiting, weakness, anxiety, and cardiac dysrhythmia.
- Hypotension is often seen in these patients.

Position

- Semi-reclined, loosen tight clothing for patient comfort.

Treatment

- Treatment of the acute coronary syndrome follows the acronym "ONAM" and begins, just like the treatment of presumed *angina*, with the administration of oxygen and nitroglycerin.
- These measures are followed by the administration of aspirin and morphine.
- The morphine provides pain relief, a feeling of euphoria, and vasodilation, which diminishes the volume of blood returning to the compromised heart.
- Nitroglycerin and oxygen dilate the coronary arteries and increase oxygen delivery, respectively, thereby reducing the area of tissue necrosis.
- The aspirin helps in preventing the platelets from aggregating, which could cause further clotting and coronary blockage.
- Sequence of treatment:
  - Activate EMS—call 911.
  - Administer O_2 by face mask.
  - Start IV.
  - Constant monitoring of vital signs.
  - If nitroglycerin has not been given already, give one dose sublingually (spray or tablet) with second dose in 5 minutes, and a third dose in another 5 minutes.
  - Morphine sulfate 1.5–3 mg increments every (q) 5 minutes.
  - Aspirin 160–325 mg tablet, chew and swallow (½ to 1 tablet).
  - Monitor for bradycardia, hypotension, dysrhythmia, and be prepared to treat.
  - Transfer to hospital.

ALLERGIC REACTION TO DRUGS

Pathophysiology

- When an allergen enters the body, certain white blood cells (plasma cells) make antibodies that attach to mast cells.
- Allergens can be virtually any foreign substance, from pollen or grass to the latex in medical gloves.
- When the same allergen enters the body again, the allergen becomes attached to two adjacent antibodies on a mast cell, and inflammatory chemicals such as histamine are released to induce profound vasodilation and bronchoconstriction.
- Mild reactions usually manifest as a skin reaction without other systemic signs or symptoms.
- *Anaphylaxis* is the most severe of allergic reactions and results from the uncontrolled release of histamine.
- Severe reactions (anaphylaxis) manifest with all signs and symptoms of allergic reaction with skin rash, watery eyes and nose, abdominal cramps, wheezing, tachycardia, and hypotension.
- Bronchoconstriction and vasodilation in anaphylaxis may trigger life-threatening dyspnea and hypotension, respectively.

Continued ▶

ALLERGIC REACTION TO DRUGS

Diagnosis

- Rash, itching, hives, swelling, sneezing, coughing, wheezing, nausea, light-headedness, and hypotension.

Position

- Horizontal (supine) or slight Trendelenburg.

Treatment

- The first and life-saving step in management of a severe allergic response is giving epinephrine.
  - Epinephrine's beta-2 (β_2) activity dilates the constricted bronchioles.
  - Its beta-2 (β_2) activity constricts blood vessels and helps control hypotension.
- Additional treatment includes administering antihistamines such as diphenhydramine (Benadryl®) to combat some of the histamine-induced components of the allergic reaction, including rashes and itching.
- In addition, a potent steroid (such as dexamethasone) is given to counteract other effects like swelling of the airway, throat, lips, and eyelids.
- Sequence of treatment for *mild reaction* (e.g., rash) usually seen > 1 hour after drug is administered:
  - Benadryl® 50–100 mg IV.
  - Follow with Benadryl® 50 mg by mouth (PO) four times daily (qid) for 2 days.
- Sequence of treatment for *severe reaction* (e.g., anaphylaxis)
  - Activate EMS—call 911.
  - Maintain chest-rising breaths with AMBU®-bag hand ventilation and, if possible, establish a fixed airway using endotracheal intubation or a laryngeal mask.
  - Administer O_2 at a flow of 4–5 L/minute.
  - Provide IV fluid if possible.
    - One liter (L) of lactated Ringer's (LR) solution is best, though normal saline or other electrolyte solutions may also suffice.
  - Administer epinephrine 1:1000 concentration, 0.3–0.5 mg subcutaneous (SQ), intra-muscular (IM) [tuberculin syringe] at 10–20 min intervals.
  - May also opt for epinephrine 1:10,000 titrated to patient response with increments of 0.2–0.5 mg IV (2–5 mL) repeated at 2–5 minute intervals as needed.
  - Benadryl® 50 mg IV: follow with Benadryl® oral dose (50 mg) for 2 days as mentioned above for mild reactions.
  - Dexamethasone 4–8 mg IV or IM.
  - Be prepared to treat:
    - Upper airway obstruction with intubation; in rare cases cricothyrotomy must be considered.
    - Hypotension.
    - Seizures.
  - Transfer to hospital and observe as an inpatient for 24 hours.

BRONCHOSPASM

Pathophysiology

- In bronchospasm, there is constriction of the terminal bronchioles that lead to the alveoli.

Continued ▶

BRONCHOSPASM

- Consequently, the flow of oxygen-containing air into the alveoli is blocked.
- This may be due to the bronchoconstriction that accompanies an allergic reaction, an asthma attack, or reaction to an irritating substance such as stomach acid in cases of aspiration.

Diagnosis

- Impairment of respiratory exchange, inspiratory and expiratory wheezes, increased resistance to ventilation, cyanosis.

Position

- Semi-reclined.

Treatment

- Treatment consists of attempting to ascertain the cause of the bronchoconstriction and removing it, accompanied by administration of a β_2 agonist, such as albuterol or epinephrine, to dilate the bronchioles and allow for passage of oxygen-bearing air into the alveoli.
- Sequence of treatment:
  - Pack surgical site and suction.
  - Activate EMS—call 911.
  - Provide positive pressure O_2.
  - Albuterol inhaler—two oral inhalations if patient is able to cooperate.
  - If patient is unconscious, support airway and apply tongue traction forward.
    - Use an extension chamber.
  - For bronchospasm not immediately responsive to inhalers, activate EMS and give epinephrine 1:1000, 0.3–0.5 mL SQ or IM.
  - Monitor for hypertension and cardiac dysrhythmia.
  - Attempt to ventilate.
  - For suspected anaphylaxis *with hypotension*:
    - Epinephrine 1:10,000 titrate to effect with 0.1–0.2 mL IV boluses up to 3–5 mL.
    - Benadryl® 50 mg/mL, 0.5–1.0 mL IV.
    - Dexamethasone 20 mg IV.
  - Monitor for dysrhythmia.
  - Transfer to hospital.

CARDIAC DYSRHYTHMIA—BRADYCARDIA

Pathophysiology

- Bradycardia is defined as a heart rate of less than 60 beats per minute.
- However, not all cases of bradycardia require treatment.
- There are many young healthy patients—especially athletes—who have resting pulses that may range from the mid-40 s to high 50 s.
- Obviously, such bradycardia does not require treatment.
- Treatment may become necessary in a medically compromised older patient who becomes symptomatic.

Diagnosis

- Pulse less than 60 is *bradycardia*, but treat the patient (and the symptoms), not the monitor.

Continued ▶

CARDIAC DYSRHYTHMIA—BRADYCARDIA

Position

• Semi-reclined, comfortable.

Treatment

• Normally there is a balance between sympathetic ("the accelerator") and parasympathetic ("the brakes") nerve supplies to the heart.
• The treatment for bradycardia is to administer atropine, which interrupts the vagal parasympathetic nerve supply, thereby "taking the foot off the brakes."
• If further rate enhancement becomes necessary, dopamine can be administered to provide sympathetic (adrenergic or adrenalin-like) stimulation, similar to "pressing the accelerator."
• Sequence of treatment:
  – Initial management:
    ○ Observe, ABCs, O_2, IV access, monitor.
  – If perfusion is adequate:
    ○ Continue to observe, ABCs, O_2, IV access, monitor.
  – If perfusion is inadequate:
    ○ If the patient demonstrates signs of (type II 2nd degree or 3rd degree) heart block, prepare for transcutaneous pacing.
    ○ Consider atropine 0.5 mg IV q 3–5 minutes to total dose of 0.03 mg/kg.
    ○ Consider dopamine 2–10 µg/minute.

CARDIAC DYSRHYTHMIA—SINUS TACHYCARDIA

Pathophysiology

• Sinus tachycardia is caused by excessive adrenergic stimulation of the sinoatrial node.
• Common causes include extreme anxiety, fever, hypovolemia, pain, exercise, hyperthyroidism, and hypoxia.

Diagnosis

• Pulse greater than 100 with a normal sinus rhythm.

Position

• Semi-reclined, comfortable.

Treatment

• Treatment for sinus tachycardia is directed at correcting the underlying problem rather than the cardiac manifestations themselves with antiarrhythmic drugs or cardioversion.
• Anxiety can be managed with a combination of patient reassurance and anxiolytics such as benzodiazepines (e.g., Valium®, Halcion®, and Versed®).
• Pain relief should be provided by local anesthetic administration and/or intravenous analgesics such as fentanyl.
• Hypoxia requires O_2 administration, a patent airway, and ventilation as needed.
• Never attempt cardioversion and avoid cardiac drugs.

EMESIS AND ASPIRATION (FOREIGN MATERIAL)

Pathophysiology

- Acid-containing gastric juices and, possibly, solid materials may be aspirated into the tracheobronchial tree.
- When the patient experiences emesis and aspirates gastric contents into the lungs, the stomach acid begins to "digest" the thin walls of the alveoli and destroy vital lung tissue.

Diagnosis

- Probable signs of vomiting (such as gagging, salivation, and coughing) followed by difficulty breathing, tachycardia, bronchospasm, cyanosis, and hypotension.

Position

- Trendelenburg, then roll patient to his/her *right* side.

Treatment

- When emesis is encountered, the patient should be placed in the Trendelenburg position and turned to his/her right side.
- The oral cavity and throat should be cleared of obstruction using finger sweeps and suction.
- If gastric contents have been aspirated, the patient should be intubated and suction performed with a catheter placed through the endotracheal tube.
- Sequence of treatment:
  - Activate EMS—call 911.
  - Clear mouth and throat with finger sweeps and large bore suction.
  - Return patient to supine position.
  - Administer muscle relaxant for rapid intubation (*to be performed only by trained personnel*).
    - If dantrolene is available, administer succinylcholine 1 mg/kg IV.
    - If dantrolene is not available, administer rocuronium 0.75–1.0 mg/kg IV.
  - Intubate with removal of foreign material as needed using Magill forceps during intubation.
  - Oxygenation and treat bronchospasm as needed using positive pressure ventilation (including continuous positive airway pressure [CPAP] if available).
  - Introduce 5–10 cc saline into endotracheal tube to facilitate suctioning and ventilate; repeat several times.
  - Do not attempt to perform tracheobronchial lavage with a large volume of fluids (*trained personnel only*).
  - Transfer to hospital.

HYPERTENSIVE CRISIS

Pathophysiology

- Markedly elevated BP constituting a hypertensive crisis usually occurs when there is excessive adrenergic or adrenaline-like stimulation.
- This leads to vasoconstriction as well as increased rate and contractile force of the heart.
- Precipitating factors can include pain, hypoxia, hypercarbia, and severe pulmonary or cardiovascular compromise (e.g., pulmonary edema).

Continued ▶

HYPERTENSIVE CRISIS

- Adrenal tumors such as pheochromocytoma may also rarely cause hypertensive episodes.

Diagnosis

- Markedly increased BP, sometimes as high as 240–250 (systolic) or 140 mm Hg and greater (diastolic).

Position

- Semi-reclined.

Treatment

- Before treatment is instituted, one should initially try to determine the cause (e.g., pain or hypoxia and hypercarbia).
- If the cause can be ascertained, possible measures should be undertaken to correct the underlying cause.
- If the BP remains elevated, it can be treated with an antiadrenergic agent such as labetalol or a vasodilator such as hydralazine.
- Sequence of treatment:
  - Stop procedure; assure patient if he/she is conscious.
  - Assess pain control, oxygenate, and then monitor electrocardiogram (EKG) to help determine etiology and concomitant conditions.
  - Treat cause, if possible.
  - If BP does not return to acceptable levels within a few minutes, administer either:
    - *Nonasthmatic patient*: Labetalol 5–20 mg IV over 2 minutes. Shorter-acting esmolol may also be used at a rate of 1 mg/kg IV, then 25–50 mg q 5 minute as needed.
    - *Asthmatic patient without cardiovascular compromise*: Hydralazine 5–25 mg IV.
    - Watch for increased heart rate and decreased BP.
  - Institute caution.
  - Do not overtreat.

HYPERVENTILATION

Pathophysiology

- Ventilation and gas exchange outpace the patient's metabolism which could lead to an excessive, unwanted exhalation of the blood bicarbonate/carbon dioxide levels.
- May be caused by the patient breathing too quickly and/or too deeply.
- Most commonly initiated by a feeling of anxiety or fear.
- Other symptoms of hyperventilation-inducing anxiety include tachycardia, chest pain, muscle stiffness, carpopedal spasm, and impaired consciousness.

Diagnosis

- Rapid breathing, anxiety, tachycardia, chest pain, muscle stiffness, carpopedal spasm, and impaired consciousness.

Position

- Semi-recumbent.

Continued ▶

HYPERVENTILATION

Treatment

- First, remove any anxiety-inducing objects that may be perceived as fearful.
- Loosen any tight clothing and reassure the patient while asking him/her to breath into the anesthesia facemask.
- The bag should be overdistended and oxygen set at approximately 0.5 L/minute.
- This builds up the CO_2 in the anesthesia bag, which triggers the proper breathing reflex control mechanisms to push respiration "back on track."
- If hyperventilation persists, consider oral anxiolytics such as Valium® 5–10 mg IV or Versed® 3 mg (3 mL)/minute up to 6 mg.
- Sequence of treatment:
  - Terminate procedure.
  - If patient is conscious, remove frightening objects such as forceps or needles from patient's line of vision.
  - If patient is conscious, remove mouth props, gauze, etc. and loosen tight clothing for patient comfort.
  - Reassure patient and talk him/her through breathing more slowly at a rate of 4–6 breaths/minute.
  - Have the patient breath into anesthesia facemask with bag overdistended and O_2 at 0.5 L/minute.
  - Alternatively, a paper bag can also help the patient rebreathe CO_2 to reset the breathing reflex.
  - If hyperventilation persists, consider diazepam (Valium®) 5–10 mg IV or midazolam (Versed®) (5 mg/mL) 2–3 mg (0.2–0.3 mL)/min IV/IM up to 6 mg.
  - Follow-up management:
    - Determine cause of anxiety.
    - Reassure the patient.

HYPOTENSION

Pathophysiology

- Hypotension is most often associated with vasodilatation.
- A large proportion of the circulating blood may become pooled in the dilated vasculatures of the abdomen and lower extremities.
- Possible etiologies include apprehension, dehydration, infection, postural change, allergic reaction, drug overdose, hypoxia, and cardiovascular compromise.

Diagnosis

- BP decreased by 20% or more; may also see loss of consciousness, weakness, nausea, tachycardia, bradycardia, or pallor.

Position

- Supine with legs above the level of the heart.
- May need to consider Trendelenburg position.

Treatment

- Initial treatment is nonpharmacologic.
- An attempt is made to determine the etiology and correct the problem if possible.

Continued ▶

HYPOTENSION

- The patient is placed in a supine or Trendelenburg position.
- A bolus of IV fluid is administered to help increase intravascular fluid levels.
- If hypotension persists, it is treated with adrenergic agents, such as ephedrine or phenylephrine, to provide cardiac stimulation and vasoconstriction.
- Sequence of treatment:
  - Stop surgery; administer 100% O_2.
  - Monitor BP, pulse (rate, rhythm, character), EKG.
  - Check level of consciousness.
  - Attempt to determine etiology: check BP, heart rate, and rhythm; and treat arrhythmia as needed.
  - Administer a bolus of IV fluids.
  - If hypotension persists, administer either:
    - Ephedrine sulfate—dilute 50 mg vial in 10 mL (5 mg/mL). Titrate to effect with 2.5–5.0 mg (0.5–1.0 mL) increments.
    - Phenylephrine HCL—dilute 10 mg from 10 mg vial 1:100. Titrate to effect with 0.1 mg (1.0 mL) increments.

INSULIN SHOCK/HYPOGLYCEMIA

Pathophysiology

- If an insulin-dependent diabetic takes his/her normal amount of insulin but has a lower intake of carbohydrates than usual (as is often the case of fasting before surgery), insulin may evacuate the already dwindling supply of glucose out of plasma and into cells.
- If the blood sugar level drops below the critical level required for brain function, the patient shows signs of low blood sugar—hypoglycemia—and could lose consciousness.

Diagnosis

- Mental clouding, lethargy followed by diaphoresis, coolness of the skin, anxiety, hypersalivation, and tachycardia.
- May lead to loss of consciousness and seizure.

Position

- Semi-recumbent.

Treatment

- Since the glucose from the blood has passed into the cells, it must be replenished with sugar taken orally or intravenously.
- An alternative is to administer glucagon, which will antagonize the actions of insulin partially by stimulating glycogenolysis (release of glucose from its storage form, glycogen) in the liver and increasing glucose levels through this route.
- Sequence of treatment:
  - Conscious patient (alert and responsive):
    - Sugar by mouth (juice, sugar water, or cola).
  - Stuporous patient:
    - Glucagon 1 mg (1 mL) IM.
    - Monitor vital signs and airway.

Continued ▶

INSULIN SHOCK/HYPOGLYCEMIA

- Unconscious patient:
  - Recline patient, support airway, monitor breathing.
  - Start IV and administer dextrose 50% 50 mL IV.
  - Monitor vital signs.
  - If unable to start IV, give glucagon as above.
  - Watch for seizures and treat as needed.
  - If consciousness does not return and the patient remains unstable, call 911.

LARYNGOSPASM

Pathophysiology

- Laryngospasm is a protective reflex that prevents foreign mater (e.g., blood, saliva, tooth fragments) from entering the larynx, trachea, and lungs.
- In a laryngospasm, the vocal cords close tightly together, inadvertently preventing the passage of oxygen-bearing air into the tracheobronchial tree.

Diagnosis

- Upon initial presentation, increased respiratory effort, decreased air exchange, supra-sternal retraction, and early "crowing" sounds can be observed.
- With a complete laryngospasm, no sound is heard.

Position

- Semi-reclined.
- Also, be prepared to place patient in Trendelenburg position.

Treatment

- An initial attempt should be made to break the laryngospasm with positive pressure O_2 via a facemask.
- If this is unsuccessful, the vocal cords can be relaxed with the muscle relaxant succinylcholine if the office has dantrolene, or rocuronium if dantrolene is not available.
- An alternative option is to deepen the anesthetic with an agent such as Propofol in an attempt to break the laryngospasm while simultaneously supporting and maintaining the airway.
- Sequence of treatment:
  - Administer 100% O_2—nasal/facemask.
  - Pack surgical site and suction.
  - Push on chest and listen.
  - Positive pressure O_2.
  - If dantrolene is available, administer succinylcholine—10 mg IV for partial laryngospasm; 20–40 mg for complete laryngospasm or barrel chest, and ventilate.
  - If dantrolene is not available, administer rocuronium 0.5 to 1 cc (5–10 mg IV) and ventilate.
    - Ventilation may be required for 15–20 min due to extended neuromuscular blockade.
    - If sugammadex is available, administer 100 mg IV to attain reversal in approximately 2–3 minutes.
  - Monitor for dysrhythmia, bradycardia, and/or pulmonary edema.

RESPIRATORY DEPRESSANT—DRUG OVERDOSE

Pathophysiology

- Patient given large dose(s) of narcotics or benzodiazepine, or even "normal" doses of these agents given for anesthesia in a patient who is overly sensitive.
- Life-threatening effects are usually due to respiratory depression as opposed to depression of the cardiovascular system.
- The primary stimulus to the respiratory centers in the brain stem that control respiration is an increase in the CO_2 level in the blood.
- Anesthetic drugs suppress the response to rising CO_2.

Diagnosis

- Decreased respiratory rate and depth (especially rate), mental clouding, and ataxia leading to loss of consciousness, pallor, and orthostatic hypotension.

Position

- Supine with legs elevated slightly or slight Trendelenburg.

Treatment

- Maintain **A**irway, **B**reathing, and **C**irculation (the ABCs) per standard Basic Life Support (BLS) protocols with airway support.
- Administer supplemental O_2.
- May need oropharyngeal or nasopharyngeal airway.
- Positive pressure ventilation may be required.
- In cases where the suspected cause is a narcotic or a benzodiazepine, antagonists like naloxone or flumazenil can be administered, respectively.
- Sequence of treatment:
  - Basic life support—maintain airway as well as monitor respiratory rate and depth.
  - O_2-assisted ventilation as needed.
  - Monitor vital signs and EKG.
  - If narcotic-induced, administer naloxone 0.4 mg IV/IM.
  - If overdose is due to a long-acting narcotic (e.g., morphine), consider an initial IV dose of 0.4 mg naloxone followed by a second IM dose of 0.4 mg as the effects of naloxone begin to wear out.
  - If benzodiazepine-induced, administer flumazenil 0.01 mg/kg up to 0.2 mg over 15 seconds.
    - This can be repeated after 45 seconds.
  - Observe patient for at least 1 hour.
  - In cases of severe overdose with the patient unstable, medical consultation and/or hospitalization should be considered.

SEIZURES

Pathophysiology

- A seizure is an abnormal electrical discharge within the brain that causes motor (i.e., muscle, sensory, or psychiatric) dysfunction, usually with loss of consciousness.
- The convulsion may be associated with an underlying seizure disorder such as epilepsy, high doses of local anesthetics containing epinephrine, and general anesthetic agents such as methohexital or ketamine, alcohol withdrawal, high fevers, or hypoglycemia.

Continued ▶

SEIZURES

Diagnosis

- Generalized (grand-mal) seizures are preceded by a prodrome of an altered emotional state, an "aura" with changes in the senses of smell, sight, and hearing, as well as widespread muscle rigidity.
- As the seizure progresses, the patient loses consciousness and emits an epileptic cry followed by muscle spasm, flailing, and possible loss of bladder and/or bowel control.
- There is a possibility of respiratory depression following the seizure.
- Etiology can include central nervous system disease, head injury, high fever, hypoxia, metabolic disorder (such as hypoglycemia), or local anesthetic overdose.

Position

- Leave patient in chair or reclining on floor.

Treatment

- The patient should be protected from injury—by ensuring that there are no dangerous objects or sharp corners nearby—but not restrained.
- A pillow can be placed beneath the patient's head and a rolled towel placed between the teeth if he/she is at risk of biting the tongue.
- For prolonged seizures greater than 5 minutes, administer diazepam (Valium®) 5–10 mg IV or IM, or midazolam (Versed®) 3 mg/min IV/IM up to 6 mg, and O_2, if possible.
  - This may help reduce the seizure intensity and/or duration.
- Monitor airway, breathing, and circulation.
- Sequence of treatment:
  - Loosen clothing, place pillow under head.
  - Do not restrain patient.
  - If patient traumatizes tongue, place rolled towel between teeth (do not use tongue blades).
  - For prolonged seizures, administer:
    - Midazolam (5 mg/mL) 2.5–5 mg (0.5–1 mL) IV/IM or diazepam 5–10 mg IV.
    - O_2 if possible
  - After seizure, support airway.
  - Continue to monitor airway, breathing, and circulation and examine mouth for injury or obstruction.
  - Suction the oropharynx if obstructions are present.

STROKE (CEREBROVASCULAR ACCIDENT)

Pathophysiology

- A stroke, or cerebrovascular accident (CVA), is an acute loss of circulation to a portion of the brain due to either occluded arteries or intracranial hemorrhage.
- When circulation to the affected area is lost, the patient develops neurologic symptoms such as paralysis, weakness, or loss of sensation on one side of the body.

Diagnosis

- Altered consciousness, hemiparesis, hemiparalysis, aphasia, headache, blurred vision, sudden hypertension greater than 140/90 mm Hg.

Continued ▶

STROKE (CEREBROVASCULAR ACCIDENT)

Position

• Comfortable, semi-upright.

Treatment

• Although definitive treatment for stroke is beyond the scope of a dentist and his/her staff, early detection and transfer to a treatment facility is essential to the patient's outcome.
• A prehospital assessment such as the Cincinnati Prehospital Stroke Scale should be performed, the ABCs followed, and the patient transferred to the appropriate facility as soon as possible.
  – Check for facial droop upon smiling.
  – Monitor drifting of the arms when they are stretched forward for 10 seconds or more.
  – Note any speech slurring.
• Sequence of treatment:
  – Terminate procedure, administer O_2, activate EMS—call 911.
  – Airway, breathing, circulation.
  – IV access and fluid bolus if patient is hypotensive.
  – Facilitate transport to hospital/stroke center as soon as possible.

SYNCOPE

Pathophysiology

• The body's response to a stressful situation is an adrenergic outflow.
• This results in shunting of blood into skeletal muscles in preparation for "fight or flight."
• However, since the patient is not actively using the musculature, the blood is not returned to the heart so that it can be recirculated to carry O_2 to the brain.
• In syncope, this can result in a temporary loss of consciousness.

Diagnosis

• Dizziness, pallor, disorientation, rapid or very slow pulse, nausea, loss of consciousness (fainting).

Position

• Supine or Trendelenburg (feet above head).

Treatment

• The patient is placed in a supine position with slight elevation of the legs.
• Provide airway support, administer O_2, and monitor.
• If there is a protracted response to repositioning, crush a vaporole of aromatic spirits of ammonia and allow the patient to breathe the vapor.
• Consider cause and treat as needed.
• Sequence of treatment:
  – Protect patient from injury.
  – Maintain airway and administer O_2.
  – Place patient in supine (or Trendelenburg) position with feet above head.
  – Monitor vital signs.
  – Consider ammonia inhalant as stimulant if the response to positioning is slow or delayed

Appendix—Helpful Terms for Understanding Medical Emergencies

- Autonomic nervous system
  - An "automatic" system that regulates most of the physiologic processes of the body.
  - The components of the autonomic nervous system keep an individual on a steady state "cruise control."
  - When the body's basic physiologic systems go awry in a medical emergency, drugs that either emulate or interfere with the autonomic nervous system are often used for treatment.
  - Consequently, crash-carts or emergency kits contain a number of these drugs.
  - For instance, epinephrine is used in cardiac arrest (asystole).
  - Adrenergic drugs such as albuterol (and epinephrine) are essential emergency medications in the treatment of asthma attacks and other allergic problems.
  - Atropine is sometimes administered in bradycardia.
- Sympathetic nervous system.
  - Adrenergic: "the accelerator."
- Parasympathetic nervous system.
  - Cholinergic: "the brakes."
- Sympathetic effects ("fight or flight").
  - Adrenergic (stimulation):
    - Alpha-1 (α-1) receptors: Found in arteries and veins and produce vasoconstriction.
    - Beta (β) receptors: Found in the "big organs" such as heart (β_1) (increase BP; increase heart rate) and lungs (β_2) (cause bronchodilation).
- Parasympathetic innervation.
  - Cholinergic:
    - Stimulates the salivary glands to produce saliva for digestion of foods.
    - Anticholinergic drugs, such as atropine or glycopyrrolate, diminish salivary secretions.
    - Normally there is a balance between the sympathetic ("the accelerator") and parasympathetic ("the brakes") nerve supply to the heart.
    - Atropine interrupts the vagal parasympathetic nerve supply, thereby "taking the foot off the brakes" and increasing the heart rate.

Bibliography

[1] Malamed SF. Medical Emergencies in the Dental Office. 6th ed. St. Louis, MO: Mosby; 2007
[2] Robert R. Emergency Preparedness. California Association of Oral and Maxillofacial Surgeons. Roseville, CA. 2017

911 CALL   Date: Time:

Pt: _____

Our Address: (type your address here)   Cross Street: _____

Our Phone #: (type your phone # here)

Patient's Age: _____   M ☐   F ☐

Type of medical emergency: _____

_____

Patient conscious? Yes ☐   No ☐ _____

Patient breathing? Yes ☐   No ☐ _____

Medications given: _____

_____

Pertinent medical history: _____

_____

Emergency treatment currently underway: _____

_____

_____

Any other questions? _____

_____

_____

Come to back door of suite – someone will be waiting to let you in.

Person making call: _____

14 Management of the Pregnant Patient

Vincent Carrao, Jeffrey A. Elo, Alan S. Herford

Introduction

Pregnancy causes many changes in the physiology of the female patient, deepening the challenges for the dental practitioner. These alterations are sometimes subtle, but can lead to disastrous complications if proper precautions are not taken. Physiologically, changes occur in the cardiovascular, hematologic, respiratory, gastrointestinal, and genitourinary systems (▶ Table 14.1).

Table 14.1 Summary of physiologic changes during pregnancy

Cardiovascular	Uterine compression of the inferior vena cava, leading to venous stasis and deep venous thrombosis
	Decreased oncotic pressure leading to lower extremity edema
	Increased red blood cell volume, heart rate
	Flattened T waves on electrocardiogram (ECG, EKG)
	Extra heart sounds (S3, systolic murmur)
	Increased cardiac output, increased plasma volume
Respiratory	Increased airway mucosa fragility leading to an increased risk of edema
	Decreased PaO_2 in supine position
	Increased risk of epistaxis with placement of nasal airway, nasogastric tube
	Progesterone-induced hyperventilation
	Decreased functional residual capacity
Hematologic	Increased risk of thromboembolic disease (hypercoagulable state)
	Leukocytosis
	Increased plasma volume creates a physiologic anemia
Gastrointestinal	Decreased lower esophageal sphincter tone leading to an increased incidence of gastroesophageal reflux disease
	Decreased gastric motility
	Increased intragastric pressure
Renal	Increased glomerular filtration rate
	Increased urinary stasis leading to urinary tract infections
	Progesterone-induced dilation of renal tree
Immune	Suppression of the maternal immune system secondary to decreased neutrophil chemotaxis, cell-mediated immunity, and natural killer cell activity

Abbreviation: PaO_2, partial pressure of oxygen.

Cardiovascular System

- Cardiac output (heart rate × stroke volume) increases 30 to 50% during pregnancy secondary to 20 to 30% increase in heart rate as well as 20 to 50% increase in stroke volume.
- Increased stroke volume is predominantly responsible for the early increase in cardiac output, possibly due to increased left ventricular mass and blood volume.
- During the second and third trimesters, a decrease in blood pressure and cardiac output can occur while the patient is in a supine position.
- This has been attributed to the decreased venous return to the heart from the compression of the inferior vena cava by the gravid uterus.
- Compression of the descending aorta can also occur, leading to decreased blood flow to the common iliac arteries.
- Hypotension, bradycardia, and syncope characterize supine hypotension syndrome.
- Not all patients become symptomatic in the supine position, but those who do may experience an initial increase in heart rate and blood pressure that soon decreases.
- While the supine pregnant patient may be asymptotic, a substantial decrease in uteroplacental perfusion can still occur.
- Placing the patient at 5 to 15% tilt on her left side can relieve supine hypotension.

Respiratory System

- An estimated 30% of all gravid patients experience symptoms of severe rhinitis.
- These changes have been attributed to the direct effects of estrogen and the indirect effects of increased blood volumes.
- Rhinitis during pregnancy appears at the beginning of the second trimester and increases in severity until delivery, then it often resolves within 48 hours.
- Mucosa in the upper airways may also become generally more edematous and friable.
- Pulmonary changes also occur in the gravid patient.
- Hyperventilation begins in the first trimester and may increase by up to 42% in late pregnancy.
- This is due in part to lower arterial carbon dioxide tension and increased renal bicarbonate excretion.
- There is also a postural effect, as well as the respiratory stimulant effects of progesterone.

- The supine position is associated with an abnormal alveolar-arterial oxygen tension gradient that significantly improves when women shift back to the sitting position.
- Approximately 50% of pregnant women complain of dyspnea by week 19 of gestation, which increases to 75% by 31 weeks.
- The dyspnea cannot be correlated with any single parameter of respiratory function; therefore, women who complain of dyspnea may only be more aware of the increased ventilation during pregnancy.
- Anatomically, the diaphragm is displaced superiorly by approximately 4 cm, which is compensated for by an increase in the transverse diameter of the thorax and the chest circumference, resulting in a 40% increase in vital capacity.
- The diaphragmatic displacement leads to 15 to 20% reduction in functional residual capacity.
- There also is a baseline 15% increase in oxygen consumption by the gravid uterus.
- These two factors result in a significant depletion in the oxygen reserve of the gravid patient.

Anesthetic and Pharmacologic Considerations

Although medications are commonly used in dental and surgical practice during pregnancy, careful consideration must be given to their effect on maternal and fetal health (▶ Table 14.2).

Local Anesthetics

- Pregnancy may affect nerve sensitivity to local anesthetics.
- Study findings have suggested a slowing of nerve conduction velocity in humans with progression of pregnancy.
- Local anesthetics freely cross the placental barrier, so the issue of fetal toxicity must be considered.
- The majority of amide type agents are bound to alpha1-acid glycoprotein.
- Pregnancy reduces alpha1-acid glycoprotein levels, resulting in increases of free local anesthetic plasma concentration and thus the potential for toxic reactions, especially with bupivacaine.
- In general, the direct effects of local anesthesia on the neonate seem to be minimal, even at higher doses.
- There are few statistically significant effects, and these are transient and so small that they likely lack clinical significance.
- The Collaborative Perinatal Project showed that the administration of benzocaine, procaine, tetracaine, and lidocaine during pregnancy did not result in an increased rate of fetal malformations.
- When local anesthesia is administered in oral surgery, it is commonly in a 1:100,000 epinephrine concentration or 10 µg/mL.

Table 14.2 Summary of commonly used medications in the dental/surgery practice and their use in pregnancy

Drug	FDA category	Use during pregnancy	During breastfeeding
Local anesthetics			
Lidocaine	B	Yes	Yes
Mepivacaine	C	Yes	Yes
Prilocaine	B	Yes	Yes
Bupivacaine	C	No, may cause hypotension	Yes
Analgesia			
Aspirin	C/D	No, associated with intrauterine growth restriction	No
Acetaminophen	B	Yes	Yes
Ibuprofen	B/C	Avoid in third trimester; may close the PDA	Yes
COX-2 inhibitor	C	Avoid in third trimester; may close the PDA	Yes
Codeine	C	Associated with first trimester malformations; can be used in second or third trimester	Yes
Oxycodone	B/C	Yes	Yes
Morphine	B	Yes	Yes
Fentanyl	B	Yes	Yes
Antibiotics			
Penicillins	B	Yes	Yes
Erythromycin	B	Yes	Yes
Clindamycin	B	Yes	Yes
Cephalosporins	B	Yes	Yes
Tetracycline	D	No	No
Sedatives			
Benzodiazepines	D	No, risk for fetal craniofacial anomalies	No
Barbiturates	D	No, risk for fetal craniofacial anomalies	No
Nitrous oxide	Not assigned	Controversial	Controversial

Abbreviation: COX, cyclooxygenase; PDA, premature ductus arteriosus.

235

- The concern in administering local anesthetic with epinephrine to pregnant patients is that the accidental intravascular injection of 15 µg of epinephrine will cause vasoconstriction of uterine arteries and decreased regional blood flow.
- In animal models, a decrease in the uterine blood flow occurs transiently, but the magnitude and duration of this decrease are equal to the decreases in uterine blood flow caused by a single uterine contraction.
- Clinically significant doses of α-adrenergic agents should be avoided to preserve placental perfusion and fetal viability.

Nitrous Oxide

- Of the anesthetic inhalation agents in use today in dentistry, the most common, and potentially the most teratogenic, is nitrous oxide (N_2O).
- The potential teratogenic effects of N_2O are related to its ability to inactivate methionine synthetase.
- Methionine synthetase is responsible for the conversion of homocysteine and methyltetrahydrofolate to methionine and tetrahydrofolate.
- Methionine is an essential amino acid and tetrahydrofolate is needed for the synthesis of DNA.
- Though there is a lack of definite clinical data in humans, there are indications that patients undergoing anesthesia with N_2O benefit from prophylactic doses of folic acid, methionine, and vitamin B_{12}.
  - A study that observed female dental assistants suggested an elevation in risk of spontaneous abortion among women who worked with nonscavenged N_2O for 3 or more hours per week.

Antibiotics

- Blood volume and creatinine clearance increase in pregnant patients that can lead to a lower serum concentration of antibiotics as compared to nonpregnant patients.
- Most antibiotics cross the placenta and thus have the potential to affect the fetus.
- Penicillin, a β-lactam structured cell wall inhibitor, has been used in clinical practice since the 1940s.
  - Of more than 3,500 fetuses included in the Collaborative Perinatal Project, there was no increase in congenital anomalies or other adverse effects after exposure to penicillin in the first trimester.
- Penicillin remains the antibiotic of choice in treating the gravid patient with an oral infection.
- Cephalosporins are the most commonly prescribed antibiotic in general use.

- Although there have been no large studies of the safety of cephalosporin use in pregnancy, teratogenic effects are yet to be reported.
- All cephalosporins, regardless of their generation, have a Food and Drug Administration (FDA) classification B, which is presumed safe based on animal models.
- The macrolide family of antibiotics is composed of erythromycin, clindamycin, azithromycin, and clarithromycin.
- Macrolides cross the placenta only minimally.
- Erythromycin and clindamycin are used extensively for oral infections in patients with allergies to penicillin or with resistant bacteria.
- All macrolides except clarithromycin are FDA class B.
  - Clarithromycin is class C, which implies an uncertain safety profile.
- The use of metronidazole in pregnancy is controversial.
  - The reduced form of the drug is teratogenic, but humans are not capable of reducing metronidazole and should not be at risk.
  - Animal models have also failed to demonstrate teratogenicity.
  - Although metronidazole has not been associated with adverse fetal effects, it is currently recommended for use in the second and third trimesters only, with an FDA classification B.
- Fluoroquinolones include norfloxacin, ciprofloxacin, ofloxacin, and enoxacin.
- There are no large epidemiologic studies of the use of fluoroquinolones in pregnancy, but these agents have shown irreversible arthropathy in immature animals.
  - Their safety during pregnancy is not established.
- Tetracyclines are bacteriostatic antibiotics that reversibly bind the 30S ribosome to inhibit bacterial protein synthesis.
- They have a very broad spectrum of coverage.
- Tetracyclines cross the placenta and deposit in fetal deciduous teeth, causing yellow-brown discoloration if given after 5 months' gestation.
- Despite earlier reports, tetracyclines do not cause enamel hypoplasia and they do not inhibit fibular growth in the preterm infant.
  - This class of medication has an overall FDA classification of D and should be avoided in pregnant patients.

Analgesics

- Codeine has been associated with fetal toxicity at below the maternal toxic doses in mice and hamster models with decreased fetal body weight.
- Codeine was not associated with an increased risk of structural malformations in mice.
- Meperidine and morphine both appear to be safe when administered for anesthesia and analgesia for short periods of time, although chronic use has been shown to cause fetal growth retardation and neonatal withdrawal.

- Nonsteroidal anti-inflammatory drugs (NSAIDs) gained popularity in the late 1970s as pain-reducing medications.
- Inhibition of prostaglandin synthesis by NSAIDs raised concerns about premature fetal ductus arteriosus constriction, which could induce primary pulmonary hypertension, closure of the premature ductus arteriosus (PDA), as well as fetal bleeding tendencies.
- Obstetricians have discouraged pregnant women from taking analgesic doses of aspirin, mainly because of the wide availability of acetaminophen.
- Fears of gastric irritation were derived from studies on patients taking large doses of aspirin and extrapolations from studies using other NSAIDs.
- Bleeding tendencies were found only in infants whose mothers had ingested 5 to 10 g of aspirin within 5 days before delivery.
  - No bleeding tendencies occurred if the aspirin was taken at least 6 days before delivery.
- Most reported cases of PDA closure occurred secondary to indomethacin administration.
- Ibuprofen, the most widely used NSAID, had no prior reports linking its use with congenital defects.
- Still, *NSAIDs should be avoided in late pregnancy because of a possibility of PDA closure.*
  - They are also classified as category C medications.

Hypnotics

- The use of benzodiazepines has shown increased incidences of cleft palate, central nervous system dysfunction, and dysmorphism in utero.
- Neurotransmitters regulate palate shelf reorientation while gamma-aminobutyric acid (GABA) inhibits reorientation.
- Benzodiazepines (diazepam specifically) may mimic GABA, thus contributing to incomplete palatal closure.

Management Modifications for the Gravid Dental Patient

- Patients may be unsure of their pregnancy status.
- If there is an uncertainty about the diagnosis of pregnancy, all treatment (unless emergent) should be postponed unless a definitive determination of pregnancy can be obtained from the patient's primary care physician.
- It is important to remember that all treatments during pregnancy are essentially rendered to two patients: the mother and the fetus.
- *All treatment should be conducted only after consultation with the patient's gynecologic specialist.*

- It is best to avoid drugs and therapy that would put a fetus at risk in all women of childbearing age for whom a negative pregnancy test has not been ensured.
- *All elective procedures should be postponed until postpartum.*
- Minor outpatient oral surgical procedures should follow basic guidelines.
- The supine position should be avoided for a variety of reasons: to avoid the development of the "supine hypotensive syndrome" in which a supine position causes a decrease in cardiac output, resulting in hypotension, syncope, and decreased uteroplacental perfusion.
- In addition, the supine position may cause a decrease in arterial oxygen tension (PaO_2) and increase the incidence of dyspepsia from gastroesophageal reflux secondary to an incompetent lower esophageal sphincter.
- Moreover, the supine position poses an increased risk of developing deep venous thrombosis by compression of the inferior vena cava, leading to venous stasis and clot formation.
- *The ideal position of the gravid patient in the dental chair is the left lateral decubitus position with the right buttock and hip elevated 15 degrees.*
- *Dental radiographs should also be kept to a minimum with appropriate patient shielding and collimation*; however, animal and human studies have shown that total exposure of more than 10 cGy radiation, or more than 5 cGy during the first trimester, is associated with intrauterine growth retardation and congenital fetal abnormalities.
- A full mouth radiographic examination exposes to 0.0001 cGy and an orthopantomogram to 0.008 cGy of radiation.
- Thus, *a minimal use of dental radiographs is acceptable for the gravid patient.*
- A computed tomography scan of the head and neck exposes to 0.01 cGy.
- The only radiographs that truly pose risks to the fetus are pelvic and abdominal films.
- *Head and neck films using a lead shield pose minimal risks to mother or fetus.*
- The use of local anesthetics in the gravid patient is acceptable, provided that uses are limited to established safe maximum doses.
- Controversy does exist regarding the use of vasoconstrictors.
  - Some practitioners avoid their use entirely, as the vasoconstrictor, usually epinephrine, introduced into vasculature may result in uteroplacental vasoconstriction with subsequent fetal hypoxia.
- Use of local anesthesia is ultimately acceptable as long as the provider exercises caution to ensure that no intravascular injection occurs.
- The use of N_2O is also controversial.
- High doses of N_2O may inhibit the enzyme methionine synthetase that in turn may hinder production of the essential amino acid methionine.
- Current guidelines dictate that N_2O use in the gravid patient is acceptable only when given at a 50% or lower mixture with oxygen.

- In addition, the patient should be given precautionary vitamins specifically to replace methionine.
- Maxillofacial infections in the pregnant patient should be addressed immediately.
- The gravid patient is more susceptible to infection for a variety of reasons.
- Hormonal changes make the mucosa more friable, with frequent chronic gingivitis.
- In addition, pregnancy has been linked to a state of mild immunosuppression.
- Nonserious infections should be managed via incision/drainage under local anesthetic with subsequent antibiotic coverage.
- It is essential to aggressively treat the gravid patient to minimize the risk of infection spreading to the fascial spaces.
- Empirical penicillin therapy is appropriate until the results of the culture/sensitivity are returned.
- More severe infections should be managed in the operating room under general anesthesia with intravenous antibiotics, and incision and drainage.

Bibliography

[1] Mabie WC, DiSessa TG, Crocker LG, Sibai BM, Arheart KL. A longitudinal study of cardiac output in normal human pregnancy. Am J Obstet Gynecol. 1994; 170(3):849–856

[2] Lee W. Cardiorespiratory alterations during normal pregnancy. Crit Care Clin. 1991; 7(4):763–775

[3] Katz VL. Physiologic changes during normal pregnancy. Curr Opin Obstet Gynecol. 1991; 3(6):750–758

[4] O'Day MP. Cardio-respiratory physiological adaptation of pregnancy. Semin Perinatol. 1997; 21(4):268–275

[5] Rosman J. Pulmonary physiology. In: ed 2. Gleicher N ed. Principles and Practice of Medical Therapy in Pregnancy. East Norwalk, CT: Appleton & Lange; 1992: 733–737

[6] Calhoun BC. Gastrointestinal disorders in pregnancy. Obstet Gynecol Clin North Am. 1992; 19(4):733–744

[7] Sevarino FB, Gilbertson LI, Gugino LD. The effect of pregnancy on the nervous system response to sensory stimulation. Anesthesiology. 1988; 69:A695

[8] Yellich GM. Perioperative considerations in the pregnant patient. Oral Maxillofac Surg Clin North Am. 1992; 4:651

[9] Axelsson G, Ahlborg G, Jr, Bodin L. Shift work, nitrous oxide exposure, and spontaneous abortion among Swedish midwives. Occup Environ Med. 1996; 53(6):374–378

[10] Rowland AS, Baird DD, Shore DL, Weinberg CR, Savitz DA, Wilcox AJ. Nitrous oxide and spontaneous abortion in female dental assistants. Am J Epidemiol. 1995; 141(6):531–538

[11] Dashe JS, Gilstrap LC, III. Antibiotic use in pregnancy. Obstet Gynecol Clin North Am. 1997; 24(3):617–629

[12] Williams J, Price CJ, Sleet RB, et al. Codeine: developmental toxicity in hamsters and mice. Fundam Appl Toxicol. 1991; 16(3):401–413

[13] Schoenfeld A, Bar Y, Merlob P, Ovadia Y. NSAIDs: maternal and fetal considerations. Am J Reprod Immunol. 1992; 28(3–4):141–147

15 Prescription Writing

Edward T. Lahey, Jeffrey A. Elo, Alan S. Herford

Introduction

- A prescription is an order for medication that is dispensed to or for an ultimate user.
  - A prescription can also be an order for a service (such as physical therapy) or medical equipment.
- To be valid, a prescription for a controlled substance must be issued for a legitimate medical purpose by a registered practitioner acting in the usual course of sound professional practice.
- Prescribing to immediate family and self-prescribing of non-controlled medications is discouraged by most licensing boards and professional associations in all but emergent situations or for very minor conditions.
- Prescribing controlled medications to immediate family or self is not allowed.
- In most states, prescription privileges for a DMD/DDS limit their prescription abilities to within their scope of dental medicine.

How to Write a Prescription

A prescription must include the following information:
- Date of issue.
- Patient's name and address.
- Practitioner's name, address, and Drug Enforcement Administration (DEA) registration number (DEA # needed for controlled substances).
- Drug name (*Rx*).
- Drug strength.
- Dosage form (tablets, capsules, liquid).
- Quantity prescribed [(*Disp*): e.g., number of tabs].
- Directions for use [(Sig): e.g., includes dosage, route of administration, frequency, and maximum dose, if relevant].
- Number of refills (if any) authorized.
- Manual signature of prescriber.

A prescription must be written in ink or indelible pencil or typewritten and must be manually signed by the practitioner.

- ▶ Table 15.1 shows commonly used prescription abbreviations.

Table 15.1 Common prescription abbreviations

Abbreviation	Meaning	Category
A.M.	Morning	Time
ac	Before meals	Time
ATC	Around the clock	Time
bid, BID	(*bis in die*) twice per day	Time
cap	Capsule	Dosage form
cc	Cubic centimeter	Measurement
disp	Dispense	Other
DOB	Date of birth	Other
g	Gram	Measurement
h, or hr	(*hora*) hour	Time
hs, or HS	(*hora somni*) at bedtime	Time
mcg	Microgram	Measurement
mg	Milligram	Measurement
mL	Milliliter	Measurement
NPO	(*nil per os*) nothing by mouth	Other
OTC	Over the counter	Other
p.r.n., or prn	(*pro re nata*) as needed	Time
pc	After meals	Time
PO, or p.o.	(*per os*) by mouth, orally	Route of administration
PM	Evening	Time
q	(*quaque*) every	Time
q4h	Every 4 hours	Time
q6h	Every 6 hours	Time
q8h	Every 8 hours	Time
qh	Every hour	Time
qhs	Each night at bedtime	Time
qid	(*quarter in die*) four times per day	Time
Rx	Prescription	Other
Sig.	(*signa*) label, let it be printed	Other
tab	Tablet	Dosage Form
tbsp	Tablespoon	Measurement
TID, tid	(*ter in die*) three times per day	Time
tsp	Teaspoon	Measurement
w/o	Without	Other
x	Multiplied by	Other

Analgesics (multimodal approach should be used)

- Recommended pain management regimen strategy that is highly effective for most patients undergoing dental procedures/dental surgery is to use alternating doses of NSAIDs and acetaminophen, with the possible addition of no more than 5–7 opioid tablets if absolutely needed for acute pain control.
  - Baseline use of *non-steroidal anti-inflammatory drugs (NSAIDs)* in combination with acetaminophen when no contraindications exist.
    - Ibuprofen 200mg: 2 tabs PO q6h prn pain; maximum 3.2g/day.
    - Acetaminophen 500mg: 2 tabs PO q6h prn pain; maximum 4g/day.
    - Each medication is dosed every 6 hours but in staggered, alternating fashion such that one or the other is taken every 3 hours.
  - On rare occasion, and only when absolutely indicated to manage acute pain, opioids may be added for moderate and severe pain not adequately controlled with NSAIDs and acetaminophen.
  - Two to three days' supply (*typically only 5–7 tabs*) is generally adequate.
  - State regulations may require:
    - Review of a patient's prescription history prior to providing a controlled substance prescription.
    - Prescribers to state that a controlled substance prescription can be partially filled.
- Mild pain.
  - Ibuprofen 200 mg: 2 tabs PO q4–6h prn pain; maximum 3.2 g/day (Ibuprofen is the GOLD STANDARD for managing post-op dental pain).
  - Acetaminophen 325 mg: 325–650 mg PO q4–6h prn pain; maximum 4 g/day.
  - Naproxen sodium 220 mg: 220–440 mg PO q8–12h prn pain; maximum 1.5 g/day.
  - Aspirin 325 mg: 325–650 mg PO q4–6h prn pain; maximum 4 g/day.
- Moderate pain (▶ Table 15.2).
  - Ibuprofen 600 mg: 1 tab PO q6h prn moderate pain; maximum 3.2 g/day (Ibuprofen is the GOLD STANDARD for managing post-op dental pain.)
  - Tylenol with codeine #3® (300 mg acetaminophen and 30 mg codeine): 1 tab PO q4–6h prn moderate pain; maximum 4 g/day acetaminophen.
  - Norco® 5/325 (5 mg hydrocodone and 325 mg acetaminophen): 1 tab PO q4–6h prn moderate pain; maximum 4 g/day acetaminophen.
  - Ultram® (tramadol 50mg): 1 tab PO q4-6h prn moderate pain; maximum 400mg/day.
  - Toradol® (ketorolac 10mg): 1 tab PO q6h prn moderate pain (this is a *non-steroidal anti-inflammatory drug [NSAID]*); maximum 40mg/day.

Table 15.2 Examples of prescriptions for moderate pain relief

Rx: Ibuprofen 600 mg	Rx: Tylenol with codeine #3®	Rx: Norco® 5/325	Rx: Ultram® 50mg
Disp: 16 (sixteen) tabs	Disp: 7 (seven) tabs	Disp: 7 (seven) tabs	Disp: 7 (seven) tabs
Sig: 1 tab PO q6h prn pain	Sig: 1 tab PO q4-6h prn pain	Sig: 1 tab PO q4-6h prn pain	Sig: 1 tab PO q6h prn pain

- Severe pain (▸ Table 15.3).
  - Norco® 7.5/325 (7.5 mg hydrocodone and 325 mg acetaminophen): 1 tab PO q4–6h prn severe pain; maximum 4 g/day acetaminophen.
  - Percocet® 5/325 (5 mg oxycodone and 325 mg acetaminophen): 1 tab PO q4–6h prn severe pain; maximum 4 g/day acetaminophen.

Table 15.3 Examples of prescriptions for severe pain relief

Rx: Norco® 7.5/325	Rx: Percocet® 5/325
Disp: 7 (seven) tabs	Disp: 7 (seven) tabs
Sig: 1 tab PO q4–6h prn pain	Sig: 1 tab PO q4-6h prn pain

- Commonly prescribed antibiotics for managing odontogenic infections (▸ Table 15.4)

Table 15.4 Examples of antibiotic prescriptions

Rx: Penicillin VK 500 mg	Rx: Amoxicillin 500 mg	Rx: Clindamycin 150 mg	Rx: Metronidazole 500 mg
Disp: #24 tabs	Disp: #18 tabs	Disp: #24 tabs	Disp: #18 tabs
Sig: 1 tab PO qid til gone	Sig: 1 tab PO tid til gone	Sig: 1 tab PO qid til gone	Sig: 1 tab PO tid til gone

- Commonly prescribed antibacterial/germicidal mouthwash for patients following oral surgery procedures (▸ Table 15.5)

Table 15.5 Example of antibacterial/germicidal mouthwash

Rx: Chlorhexidine gluconate 0.12%

Disp: 473 mL (one bottle)

Sig: 15 mL PO swish 30 second/spit bid until gone

Index